Colon & Rectal Cancer

From Diagnosis to Treatment

Second Edition

Paul Ruggieri, M.D.
Addison R. Tolentino, M.D.

Addicus Books
Omaha, Nebraska

An Addicus Nonfiction Book

ISBN 978-1-886039-05-6

Cover and interior design by Jack Kusler
Illustrations by Jack Kusler

This book is not intended to serve as a substitute for a physician, nor do the authors intend to give medical advice contrary to that of an attending physician.

Library of Congress Cataloging-in-Publication Data

Ruggieri, Paul, 1959-
   Colon & rectal cancer : from diagnosis to treatment / Paul
Ruggieri, Addison R. Tolentino. -- 2nd ed.
      p. cm.
   Includes bibliographical references and index.
   ISBN 978-1-886039-05-6 (pbk.)
1. Colon (Anatomy)--Cancer. 2. Rectum--Cancer. I. Tolentino,
Addison R., 1969- II. Title. III. Title: Colon and rectal cancer.
 RC280.C6R84 2011
 616.99'4347--dc23

                                                    2011031606

                        Addicus Books, Inc.
                          P.O. Box 45327
                       Omaha, Nebraska 68145
                       www.AddicusBooks.com

               Printed in the United States of America
                   10 9 8 7 6 5 4 3 2 1

Contents

Acknowledgments

I would first like to thank all my patients, past and present, for the privilege of being involved in their care. I would also like to acknowledge my patients' family members. Their love, understanding, and support are so vital to a loved one's recovery.

I would like to thank Christine Gillespie, R.N., both for her care of my colorectal cancer patients and for her input in this book. I wish to thank Diane Peckham, R.N., certified wound, ostomy, and continence nurse, for her expertise on the care of a colostomy.

I wish to thank radiation oncologist Carol Kornmehl, M.D., author of *The Best News about Radiation Therapy*, for her contribution to the chapter on radiation therapy. I would also like to thank Mark Pool, M.D., Laboratory Medical Director at Riverside Medical Center, Kankakee, Illinois, for his help in the development of this book.

This book would not have been possible without the efforts of all those involved at Addicus Books. I especially thank Rod Colvin for his uncompromising focus and drive for perfection. I also express my appreciation to Jack Kusler for his illustrations and design work.

Finally, I would like to thank Larry Connors for his inspiration, and my parents for their courage and support.

Paul Ruggieri, M.D.

Several people made it possible for me to coauthor this book. I would like to acknowledge them all. First, I thank Kris Gaster for introducing me to Addicus Books and the opportunity to be part of the book.

I thank Jessica Muth, nutritionist at the Avera Cancer Institute, for providing information about nutrition during chemotherapy; her contribution was most helpful. I also thank my team, Michelle, Jill, and, Steph, at the Avera Cancer Institute, for their ongoing support.

I wish to thank my family. To my wife, Keesha, and my daughter, Aliyah, I appreciate your love and support during the time I spent working on this book. I also acknowledge my parents. I am grateful to them for having sent me to medical school. Without their love and support, I would not be doing the work of a physician—work that fulfills me on a daily basis.

I express my appreciation to my publisher Rod Colvin at Addicus Books. A wise adviser, he worked patiently and diligently with me, stressing the importance of clarity and simplicity in the text so that we could do the best job possible in serving readers.

Finally, I thank my patients, who have taught me so much during my years as a medical oncologist. I dedicate this book to you.

Addison R. Tolentino, M.D.

Introduction

Has your life suddenly been interrupted by an unexpected diagnosis of colon or rectal cancer? Or, has someone close to you just been diagnosed with the disease? If so, your first reaction may be shock, denial, or anger. It doesn't seem fair that you're suddenly forced to come face-to-face with a life-threatening disease. You may be thinking, Why me? Why my family? Your reactions and feelings are normal and understandable. It may be of comfort to know that you are not alone.

Unfortunately, cancer affects nearly everyone directly or indirectly. If you or an immediate family member has not been diagnosed with it, you probably know someone who has. This is especially true of colorectal cancer. Colorectal cancer is the third most common cancer in the United States, and the third leading cause of cancer death in the United States.

Our goal in writing this book is to provide you with some peace of mind by answering those pressing questions that arise with a diagnosis of cancer. It is our hope that this book will serve as your guide as you make the journey through treatment.

1 Colorectal Cancer: An Overview

It seems nothing can prepare us for a diagnosis of cancer. Being told you have cancer can bring on a flood of emotions—shock, fear, and confusion. At first, it may be difficult to comprehend the fact that you have cancer. And, in addition to coming to grips with the diagnosis, you're faced with undergoing medical tests and a series of treatments, all of which you probably know little about. It can be a stressful time for you, your family, and friends.

The term "colorectal cancer" actually refers to two diseases. Colon cancer is cancer found in the tissues of the colon, and rectal cancer forms in the tissues of the rectum. Both cancers have the same characteristics and the same risk factors. In some cases, they are treated the same way, while at other times the treatments are different.

Colorectal Cancer Statistics

Not counting skin cancer, colon cancer is the third most commonly diagnosed cancer in the United States. It affects approximately 102,000 Americans each year, according to the American Cancer Society. Rectal cancer is less common than colon cancer, affecting nearly 40,000 people annually. Both cancers are curable if detected early. And, thanks to improved treatments and greater public awareness about preventive screening, death rates from colorectal cancer have been dropping over the last twenty years.

Anatomy and Function of the Colon and Rectum

Before discussing colorectal cancer and how it develops, let's first take a brief look at the anatomy of the colon and rectum. The colon and rectum are important parts of your *gastrointestinal (GI) tract.* This tract includes your mouth, *esophagus,* stomach, *duodenum* (first part of your small intestine), small intestine, colon (large intestine), rectum, and anus. This system takes in food, digests it, absorbs nutrients, and excretes waste.

The primary job of the colon is to manage and remove solid waste. When you eat, food spends several hours in the stomach being digested. Once the nutrients are absorbed in the small intestine, any remaining liquid enters the colon, which is also called the large bowel.

By the time the liquid enters the first part of the colon, it contains no nutrients and is pure waste product. This waste liquid is slowly propelled toward the rectum. Over a four- to six-hour period, the cells in the colon absorb remaining water from the waste material. The colon can absorb nearly two gallons of water a day. The end product is the solid waste, or feces.

The rectum's primary function is to store processed fecal material before it is excreted from the body. Once there is enough fecal material in the rectum, sensory nerves tell the brain it is time to have a bowel movement.

Colorectal Cancer in the U.S.

- Colon cancer cases diagnosed annually:
  Women: 53,000
  Men: 49,000

- Rectal cancer cases diagnosed annually:
  Men: 23,000
  Women: 17,000

- Approximately 72% of cases are colon cancer.

- Approximately 28% of cases are rectal cancer.

- Lifetime chances of developing colorectal cancer: 1 in 20

American Cancer Society

Frontal View of Colon

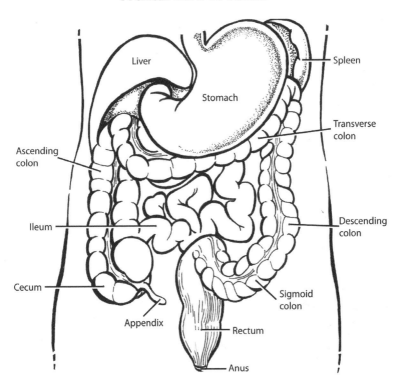

The Colon

The colon is a hollow, tubelike organ that is five to six feet long and up to five inches in diameter. It sits in the abdominal cavity and is divided into segments. The first segment is the *cecum,* which is a pouch that receives waste material from the small intestine. The next segment is the *right (ascending) colon,* located on the right side of the abdomen. The *transverse colon* crosses over the midsection of the abdomen. The *left (descending) colon* is on the left side of the abdominal cavity. The left colon leads into the *sigmoid colon,* an S-shaped section that connects to the rectum. The rectum is a muscular tube, the last six to ten inches of the colon, and it exits into the anus.

3

The colon itself has four layers of tissue. The innermost layer, the *mucosa*, is in direct contact with fecal material moving through the colon and is responsible for much of the colon's function. The thin mucosa is composed of specialized cells that are in a constant state of flux, continually dying, sloughing off, and being replaced with new cells. The layer under the mucosa is the *submucosa*. It's a specialized layer of cells that helps support the mucosa.

The next layer of tissue is the *muscularis propria*. The muscle cells in this layer give strength to the colon wall and cause the contractions that push fecal material along the colon. The outermost layer of tissue is the *serosa*. The serosal cells add more support to the colon wall and act as a barrier, protecting the colon from any outside invading disease.

The Rectum

The rectum, the last six to ten inches of the colon, connects the colon to the anus. Unlike the rest of the colon, the walls of the rectum are primarily composed of muscle cells that propel the fecal material out of the body.

The last part of the digestive system is the anus. It is a canal, about two inches long, that contains sphincter muscles; it's the job of these muscles to hold in waste material until you're ready to have a bowel movement.

How Colorectal Cancer Develops

Colorectal cancer usually develops from *polyps*, which are small, abnormal growths that can occur anywhere along the gastrointestinal tract. Polyps are common in the colon and rectum; in fact, as many as 50 percent of the U.S. population has polyps in the colon and/or rectum. Polyps occur more frequently in people over age fifty; they are caused by genetic changes in the cells lining the inside of the colon and grow slowly over a period of ten to fifteen years. Cancer is an overgrowth of these abnormal cells and, sometimes, polyps start growing uncontrollably. Most people have no idea a tumor is growing inside their colon or rectum unless they go for routine tests or start to experience symptoms such as pain or bleeding.

Types of Polyps

Colorectal polyps may be benign or malignant (cancerous). Fortunately, most polyps are benign. Only about 1 percent of polyps that are removed prove to be cancerous. Still, it's important to know that benign polyps can turn into cancer if not removed.

Benign Polyps

Polyps referred to as benign are noncancerous. Several types of benign polyps may occur in the colon. The polyps are defined by their size and the appearance of their cells under the microscope.

- *Hyperplastic.* About 90 percent of all polyps are hyperplastic polyps. They are small, about the size of a pea, and consist of a dense cluster of normal cells with no microscopic abnormalities. They are totally benign, with no potential to become cancerous.
- *Inflammatory.* This type of benign polyp, also small, is made up of inflamed cells commonly associated with inflammatory diseases of the colon, including ulcerative colitis and Crohn's disease.
- *Hamartoma.* This type of small, benign polyp is found in patients with genetically inherited polyp syndromes. (See discussion of these syndromes later in this chapter.) These polyps are frequently numerous and scattered throughout the colon.

Precancerous Polyps

A polyp can also be labeled *precancerous.* This means the growth contains suspicious-looking cells when viewed under the microscope, but these cells do not yet meet the criteria to be called malignant. If precancerous cells are not removed or treated, they can develop into cancer that can spread. These polyps are divided into three categories.

- *Tubular.* This type of polyp may be found anywhere in the colon. Most are about one-fourth inch in diameter but may grow to three-fourths inch. They are made up of cells that are tubular in shape. Tubular polyps are generally considered premalignant with a 5 percent chance of becoming cancerous if not removed.

- *Tubulovillous.* This type of polyp typically grows to about one-half inch in diameter and has a cluster of finger-like projections. These polyps have a higher potential—20 percent—to turn into cancer.

- *Villous.* These premalignant polyps are often found in the rectal area; they can grow to one to two inches in diameter. Villous polyps have the greatest potential— up to a 40 percent chance—to become malignant.

Cancerous Polyps

When a polyp is found to be cancerous, the cancer may be classified as *carcinoma in situ* or as *adenocarcinoma.*

- *Carcinoma in situ.* These polyps contain cancer cells that are at the beginning of their life cycle. The malignant cells are contained within the polyp and do not spread to other organs.

- *Adenocarcinoma.* These cancerous polyps have the potential to spread outside the polyp to other organs. This type of cancer is the most common form of colorectal cancer, making up nearly 96 percent of all cases.

Characteristics of Cancerous Polyps

Several factors influence whether a colorectal polyp is malignant. These factors include the size of the polyp, its shape, location, in the colon, and the presence or absence of microscopic changes to the DNA, the cell's blueprint for growth.

Size

The larger the polyp, the greater the chance of it being cancerous. For instance, a polyp less than one-half inch in diameter has a less than 10 percent chance of being cancerous. However, polyps more than one inch in diameter can have a 20 to 30 percent chance of being cancerous. It is important to remove polyps early so they cannot grow to sizes that increase the potential for cancer.

Shape

The general shape of a colorectal polyp also influences the potential of it being cancerous. Polyps that are located on a "stalk," with the stalk attached to the inner lining of the colon wall, are easily removed and less likely to be cancerous. However, polyps that are very broad based are more difficult to remove and more likely to be cancerous. Broad-based polyps are called *sessile polyps.*

Examples of the polyps on a "stalk" are shown above. These polyps are less likely to be cancerous.

Broad-based, or sessile, polyps, are more likely to be cancerous.

Location

The location of a polyp is also important. Cancerous polyps are more commonly found in the sigmoid colon and rectum than in other parts of the colon. It has been estimated that more than 50 percent of cancerous polyps are located in the sigmoid colon and rectum; the sigmoid is the part of the large intestine that is closest to the rectum and anus.

Dysplasia

Dysplasia is the medical term used to describe the genetic mutations (abnormalities) observed in the DNA of polyp cells. When cells are dysplastic their centers (*nuclei*) are misshapen. The more dysplastic changes, the greater the chance of finding cancer cells. Dysplastic changes can lead to cancerous tumors.

Symptoms of Colorectal Cancer

Early on, the symptoms of colorectal cancer often go unnoticed. You may feel fine, with no indication of any problem. Fortunately, routine screening often leads to the detection of colorectal cancer even when you have no symptoms.

By the time symptoms are obvious, colorectal cancer has often progressed. Unfortunately, many people ignore the signs and do not report them to their doctor. Some people do not realize that a change in bowel habits or blood in the stool may be a sign of cancer. Other people are embarrassed to talk about such symptoms. However, ignoring such symptoms may delay the early diagnosis of a potentially curable cancer.

Fatigue

Fatigue has many causes and is not always a symptom of colorectal cancer. However, when fatigue is caused by iron deficiency anemia, it may be a symptom of colorectal cancer. This anemia is caused by the body's not receiving enough iron to produce healthy *red blood cells*, which carry oxygen to the body's other cells. Such anemia could be the result of the slow, progressive loss of blood caused by a tumor. You may not notice the anemia right away, but it can lead to noticeable symptoms such as fatigue, pale appearance, dizziness, or shortness of breath during physical activity.

Change in Bowel Habits

A common early-warning symptom of colorectal cancer is a subtle change in your bowel habits. Changes in your bowel pattern may include:

- Persistent loose stools.
- Constipation.
- Vague discomfort with bowel movements.
- Changes in the shape of stools, such as pencil-thin stools.
- A painful urge to have a bowel movement when it's not needed. This urge or feeling of incomplete evacuation of the bowels is known as *tenesmus*. It may be caused by a tumor growing inside the rectum that takes up space and creates pressure.

Rectal Bleeding

Passing bright red or dark blood is another warning symptom of colorectal cancer. The bleeding may be coming from a polyp or a cancer. You may notice blood on toilet paper or blood mixed in with a bowel movement; if the blood is mixed with stool, it may be dark, almost black, in color.

Passing blood may occur without pain. You may not even notice it if the blood loss is subtle and occurs slowly. It is possible that rectal bleeding could be caused by a hemorrhoid; however, it's important to report any rectal bleeding to your physician.

Abdominal Pain or Bloating

Abdominal pain is not a common warning symptom for colorectal cancer during its early stages. However, if the disease has spread beyond the colon or rectal wall into other organs, abdominal cramping and pain may occur. Individuals with this type of abdominal pain usually describe it as a dull, nagging, intermittent pain that does not go away with the use of over-the-counter antacids. Unfortunately, many people ignore such pain until it starts to impact their everyday activities. If you have recurrent pain, do not attribute it to an upset stomach, stress, or food choices. If the cancer should cause a perforation in the colon, the pain will likely worsen and may require a visit

---

**Symptoms of
Colorectal Cancer**

• Fatigue caused by iron
  deficiency anemia

• Change in bowel habits

• Rectal bleeding

• Chronic abdominal pain,
  bloating, or fullness

• Painful urge to have a bowel
  movement

• Decreased appetite or
  unintended weight loss

---

to an emergency room.

Other times, people may not feel pain, but will report feeling full after eating very little. If cancer has spread to the inner lining of the abdominal cavity, an accumulation of fluid may result. This may cause bloating or rapid distension of the belly. Sometimes, people say they can feel a mass in their abdomen that was never there before.

If you experience any of these symptoms, see your doctor.

Decreased Appetite, or Unintended Weight Loss

Some people with colorectal cancer complain of not having an appetite or of losing weight despite eating. It's possible that appetite could be affected by a tumor or fluid in the abdomen, causing you to feel full after eating very little. The reason that having cancer may cause weight loss is complex and not totally understood. It is believed that when you have cancer, the body releases destructive proteins, which leads to an increased metabolic rate, that is too high for sustaining body weight. Your body may not be absorbing all the fat, protein, and carbohydrates from the food you eat. Or your body may be burning calories faster than normal. The result is weight loss.

Bacterial Infection

Sometimes, colorectal cancer will cause an abscess in the abdomen. Bacteria that reside in the colon can escape through the abscess and into the bloodstream. Having an infection in the bloodstream is a serious, life-threatening condition. It is referred to as *bacteremia*, or *sepsis*. Symptoms include chills, fever, drop in blood pressure, rapid heart rate, hyperventilation, light-headedness, and confusion. This condition requires emergency medical care.

Stroke-like Symptoms

Symptoms similar to those of a stroke are rarely the first symptoms of colorectal cancer. However, it is possible that some colorectal cancers may go undetected until the cancer has spread to parts of the brain. Symptoms would include stroke-like symptoms, such as weakness or numbness in the face, arm, or leg. Other possible symptoms are blurred vision, slurred speech, and seizures.

Risk Factors for Colorectal Cancer

What are the risks for developing colorectal cancer? No one knows exactly what causes colorectal cancer. However, doctors think genetic changes, coupled with dietary and environmental factors, play a role in normal cells changing into cancerous cells.

The following risk factors increase the chances for developing colorectal cancer sometime in your life. Fortunately, some of the risks are related to lifestyle, and making changes in lifestyle can decrease your risk.

Family History

A family history of colorectal cancer is the most important risk factor. According to the National Cancer Institute, 25 percent of individuals diagnosed with colon cancer have a family history of the disease. Having someone in your family with colorectal cancer, particularly a parent or sibling, puts you at a much higher risk than someone without a family history of the disease. If a relative such as an aunt, uncle, or cousin has had colorectal cancer, the risk is lower, but still higher than for those with no family history of the disease.

Several genetically inherited syndromes may predispose

you to developing early colorectal cancer. If you or a member of your family is diagnosed with one of these syndromes, you're at higher risk. Fortunately, most of these syndromes are rare. However, they can be deadly if not diagnosed and treated early.

Hereditary nonpolyposis colon cancer (HNPCC), also known as *Lynch syndrome*, accounts for about 5 percent of all colon cancers. It causes the formation of one to five potentially cancerous polyps in people in their thirties or forties; however, the polyps can also occur earlier, before age twenty. Individuals with this syndrome have an 80 percent chance of developing colon cancer at some point in their lives.

Families with this abnormal gene usually have three or more closely related family members who have   been diagnosed with colorectal cancer, colon cancer affecting family members in two generations, and at least one family member who has been diagnosed with colorectal cancer before the age of fifty.

Familial adenomatous polyposis (FAP) is a rare, inherited disease that causes the formation of hundreds or even thousands of polyps along the gastrointestinal tract. These polyps typically form during the teenage years and, if left untreated, will nearly always turn cancerous by the time the person reaches his or her late thirties. This syndrome is mostly associated with polyps in the colon, but may affect other organs, such as the liver, thyroid gland, and brain.

Gardner's syndrome is another rare disease. A variation of FAP, it can cause hundreds of polyps in the colon or small intestine; it may also cause benign tumors in the skin, bone, or abdomen.

Turcot's syndrome is a rare, inherited disorder in which multiple polyps form in the colon, causing an increased risk for colon cancer. There is also a risk of cancer developing in the brain.

Peutz-Jeghers syndrome is a condition marked by the development of freckles all over the body. Polyps, which may become malignant, form in the colon.

Cowden's syndrome is a rare disorder that causes benign tumors in the skin and mucous membranes of the mouth and nose. However, polyps may form in the colon, increasing the risk for colon cancer.

Finally, there is also increasing evidence that a family history of uterine, breast, or ovarian cancer may increase the risk for colorectal cancer. Knowing your family history is important to understanding your risk and developing a screening plan with your doctor.

Age

Anyone at any age can develop colorectal cancer. However, more than 90 percent of the people diagnosed with colorectal cancer are over the age of fifty. The average age of people diagnosed with colorectal cancer is close to seventy. If you're under age forty and have no other risk factors, you're at very low risk for getting colorectal cancer. After age fifty, however, population studies show that your risk increases dramatically. That's why routine checkups and screening for most people should start at age fifty.

Medical History

If you have had colorectal polyps or have been treated for colorectal cancer in the past, you are at a much higher risk for redeveloping either disease in the future. Follow-up tests after you have been treated for colorectal cancer are critical.

Diet

What you eat affects your risk. A diet high in meat and saturated fats and low in fiber (the so-called Western diet) places you at greater risk for developing colorectal cancer.

This is evident in studies of Japanese immigrants to the United States. The incidence of colorectal cancer in Japan is much lower than in the United States. This is presumably due to the high-fiber, low-fat diet prevalent in Japan. However, when

Japanese come to the United States and adopt a more Western diet, within two generations their risk of developing colorectal cancer is the same as that of Americans.

The risk stems from potential cancer-causing agents, or *carcinogens*, that can form when the body ingests fatty acids and cholesterol. When fatty foods are cooked and processed, saturated fatty acids and cholesterol are broken down into potential cancer-causing by-products. Over time, these carcinogens interact with the cells lining the inside of the colon, damaging their DNA. The damaged (mutated) DNA can then greatly increase the potential of these cells to turn cancerous.

It is well known that a diet high in fiber can reduce the risk for many diseases affecting the colon, including cancer. Fiber is thought to trap or dilute the cancer-causing agents in our diet. Fiber also flushes out these agents quickly, decreasing the time they are in contact with the lining of the colon.

Inflammatory Bowel Diseases

Two *inflammatory bowel diseases* that affect the lining of the colon are associated with an increased risk of colorectal cancer over time. These diseases are *ulcerative colitis* and *Crohn's disease*.

Ulcerative colitis causes inflammation of the inner layer of colon cells and results in chronic pain, bleeding, and diarrhea. It can affect an isolated segment of the colon or the entire organ. The cause of ulcerative colitis is not known, and there is no effective medical cure. Surgery often is the only potential curative option, but it can't prevent the disease from coming back later in life. During the first ten years that a person has ulcerative colitis, the risk of developing colorectal cancer is low. However, after the first ten years, the risk increases 20 percent every ten years. Routine screening should begin after the initial diagnosis.

Crohn's disease also increases the risk for colorectal cancer. Like ulcerative colitis, Crohn's disease involves inflammation of the inner layer of the colon. It usually also involves other layers of the colon wall. Crohn's disease leads to abdominal pain, bleeding, infection, blockages, and diarrhea. The disease has no known cause, and treatment can be difficult. The longer a person lives with Crohn's disease, the greater the risk for developing colorectal cancer.

Smoking

Studies by the American Cancer Society show that prolonged smoking can significantly increase your risk of colorectal cancer. According to the data, if you have smoked for more than twenty years, your risk of dying from colorectal cancer increases 40 percent. Clearly, the more you smoke, the more you increase your risk of cancer. It is also evident that the younger you start smoking, the greater your risk. This is true for both men and women.

Obesity and Physical Inactivity

Several medical studies indicate that being overweight and physically inactive increases the risk for colorectal cancer. If you're very overweight—especially if you carry your excess weight around your waist—you're at even greater risk for colorectal cancer. Some research suggests that excess fat changes metabolism (how the body converts food to energy) in a way that increases the growth of cells in the colon.

People who don't get a minimum amount of exercise are also at increased risk for colorectal cancer. Studies suggest that exercise, such as jogging or walking, may lower the risk for colorectal cancer. Exercise also has well-known benefits for the heart and lungs and helps control weight.

Exposure to Asbestos

Some studies show an increased risk of colorectal cancer for workers who have had contact with asbestos, the fibrous material once used in insulation for residential and commercial construction. The Agency for Toxic Substances and Disease Registry (ATSDR) agrees that some studies show a link between asbestos exposure and colorectal cancer; however, the agency says there is no definitive proof that exposure to asbestos causes colorectal cancer.

In Summary

We've discussed some of the potential causes of colon and rectal cancer along with symptoms. If you had these symptoms, you may have already undergone diagnostic testing. Or, perhaps you are scheduled for tests. The next chapter discusses the medical tests that are commonly used to diagnose colon and rectal cancer.

2 Getting a Diagnosis

Getting colorectal cancer diagnosed early might mean the difference between curing the cancer and discovering that the cancer has advanced. The five-year survival rate for people who are diagnosed and treated early is 90 percent.

It takes five to ten years for colon cancer to grow through the colon wall; hopefully this expanse of time will increase the likelihood that an individual will have a colon cancer screening test or seek medical attention for symptoms. Still, doctors cannot predict which cancers will spread. Some smaller tumors may, for reasons not fully known, release cancer cells into the bloodstream, allowing them to spread to other organs. Other times, tumors may grow to a large size but not spread.

About 37 percent of colorectal cancers are detected early, before any spread has occurred. However, approximately 37 percent of the time, the cancer has spread to surrounding tissues. In about 20 percent of cases, the cancer has spread to distant organs.

Medical History and Physical Examination

During a visit to your doctor, he or she will take a personal and medical history and ask you about your symptoms. The doctor will ask about any changes in your bowel habits, passing of blood, abdominal pain, weight loss, and/or decreased appetite. The doctor will also want to know if you have any family history of colorectal cancer, including which relatives may have had colon cancer and their ages at the time of diagnosis. A complete and accurate personal and family medical history can provide your doctor with important clues that can help diagnose your condition.

Your physician will also likely perform a thorough physical examination. He or she will observe whether you're pale, which can be a sign of anemia, a deficiency in red blood cells. The doctor will perform a digital exam of your rectum, checking for possible masses; the doctor will also examine your abdomen to detect any bloating or masses. However, if cancer is just starting, the doctor may not find anything abnormal during the initial exam.

Diagnostic Tests

If colorectal cancer is suspected, your physician will schedule you for diagnostic testing. He or she may do the initial testing and then may refer you to specialists for additional testing.

Fecal Occult Blood Test (FOBT)

The *fecal occult blood test (FOBT)* is used to find occult (hidden) blood in your feces. The screening involves placing a smear of stool on a card and applying a drop of a liquid chemical onto the feces. If a trace amount of blood is present in your stool, the card turns blue, a positive test result. Only 2 to 4 percent of patients tested will be found to have a positive test for fecal occult blood.

A positive FOBT result does *not* necessarily mean you have colorectal cancer. It means your doctor needs to perform additional tests to find the source of the blood. One negative aspect of the fecal occult blood test is its accuracy. The test is not very specific for the presence of colorectal cancer. There are many other diseases of the colon, including hemorrhoids, rectal ulcers, fissures, Crohn's disease, ulcerative colitis, *diverticulosis*, polyps, and trauma from the exam itself that can cause you to have a positive test result. Despite not being very specific, the fecal occult blood test is simple, cost-effective, and helpful in beginning the process of detecting colorectal cancer.

Stool DNA Test

A newer test, the *stool DNA test* is similar to the fecal occult blood test, which looks for blood in the stool. However, the stool DNA test is used to check for both blood and abnormal genetic materials from polyps or cancer cells. Polyps and colon cancers are continually shedding DNA cells that will eventually show up in the stool.

The test is not invasive and requires no preparation to clean out the colon. It does require the collection of an entire stool sample. Typically, patients are given special kits for collecting the sample, which must reach the laboratory within twenty-four hours. This test is not used widely because of the need for the entire stool sample and because it is more expensive to test the DNA.

Colonoscopy

A *colonoscopy* is considered the best diagnostic test for colorectal cancer. It is the most effective way to evaluate the inside of your entire colon for the presence of polyps or cancer. Because the colonoscope has wire snares and biopsy forceps, a doctor can also remove any polyps that are found and can biopsy or even remove a tumor. Performed in an outpatient setting, at a hospital or surgery center, the procedure is performed by either a gastroenterologist or a general surgeon.

Your colon must be empty and clean before the procedure. This usually involves drinking a liquid laxative and avoiding solid foods the day before; you'll be allowed to drink only clear liquids. Before undergoing a colonoscopy, you'll be given light sedation since the procedure can cause some discomfort as the colonoscope is guided through the colon.

To perform the procedure, the physician gradually advances a flexible fiber-optic scope through the entire colon. Air inflates the colon so the doctor can have a clear view of the entire colon lining on a television monitor. The procedure takes approximately thirty minutes.

Afterward, you'll be taken to a recovery area and monitored by nurses until you're awake. You'll need to have someone take you to the procedure and pick you up afterward. Typically, before you leave, your doctor will let you know whether any polyps or tumors were detected. If either is found, laboratory tests will be performed on the tissues to determine whether cancer is present.

Colonoscopy is safe, but not totally risk free. Possible complications include bleeding after polyp removal, and perforation of the colon. Perforation of the colon is rare, occurring 0.2 to 0.4 percent of the time; this complication, however, does require emergency surgery to repair. In addition, potential adverse reactions to the intravenous sedation include nausea, vomiting, and temporary breathing distress.

About 10 to 20 percent of the time, the physician is unable to view the entire colon successfully. This may be a result of incomplete bowel cleansing the day before, or the doctor may not be able to navigate all the turns in the colon. When this occurs, a follow-up barium enema may be necessary to complete the examination.

Flexible Sigmoidoscopy

The *flexible sigmoidoscopy* is a test that allows a doctor to check for polyps or cancer in the lower part of the intestine, where nearly 50 percent of all colorectal cancer occurs.

The sigmoidoscope is a thin, flexible fiber-optic tube that contains a tiny camera at the tip. The tube, about thirty inches long, is connected to a television monitor, allowing the doctor to examine the last several feet of the colon (sigmoid colon) and the entire rectum. The procedure is carried out in the doctor's office and takes about ten minutes. No anesthesia is necessary since the procedure isn't painful. The procedure may be performed by your primary care doctor, an internist, a general surgeon, or a gastroenterologist, who is a physician trained in diagnosing and treating diseases of the colon.

During a sigmoidoscopy, as the scope is inserted into the anus and directed into the rectum, you'll feel a slight pressure sensation as air is pumped through the scope and into the colon. The air expands the inside of the colon so the doctor can examine the entire lining. If a polyp or tumor is discovered, it can be removed with the sigmoidoscope for laboratory examination.

If your doctor orders a sigmoidoscopy, you'll be instructed to give yourself an enema the night before the procedures to cleanse your bowels. You'll need to avoid food and beverages on the morning of the procedure; however, your doctor will likely tell you it's okay to take medications with water.

Colonoscopy

A colonoscopy is performed to examine the entire colon for polyps or cancer.

Sigmoidoscopy

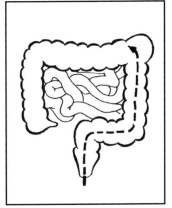

A sigmoidoscopy is performed to examine the lower portion of the colon.

The flexible sigmoidoscopy has several advantages: It can be performed in five to fifteen minutes in a doctor's office; it usually does not cause discomfort; and it carries less risk for complications than a colonoscopy.

The disadvantage is that since it is used to examine only the lower part of the colon, it can miss polyps and cancers in other parts of the colon. Studies have shown that if your screening flexible sigmoidoscopy is normal, there is up to a 3 percent chance you could still have a cancer in the side of your colon not reached by the sigmoidscope.

Possible complications of sigmoidoscopy include perforation of the colon or rectum by the scope. These complications are rare, however, occurring in only 1 out of 10,000 procedures. However, if a perforation does occur, emergency surgery is needed to repair the perforation.

Computerized Tomography (CT) Colonography

Another test used to examine the colon is the *computerized tomography (CT) colonography*, also known as a *virtual colonoscopy*. In this procedure, a scope is not inserted through the rectum. Instead, you are placed inside a sophisticated computerized tomography (CT or CAT) scanner; the scan provides detailed two- and three-dimensional images of your colon.

The procedure has several advantages: It is less invasive and less uncomfortable than a standard colonoscopy; it can be done in about ten minutes; and it does not require sedation. However, a rubber tube used to insert air into the colon to expand it is still needed. The bowel cleansing preparation is also the same as for other tests using a scope. If a polyp is found on a virtual colonoscopy, you will still need a standard colonoscopy to have it removed.

Double-Contrast Barium Enema

If your doctor decides your entire colon needs evaluation,

he or she may order a *double-contrast barium enema,* which may be done at the same time as a flexible sigmoidoscopy. During the procedure, air and barium, a white liquid (contrast), are injected into the bowels through a tube that is inserted in the rectum. Several X-rays are taken and then read by a *radiologist,* a doctor trained in reading X-rays. The procedure takes an hour and is performed on an outpatient basis in the radiology department of a hospital or surgery center. Although this test isn't painful, most people experience a sensation of pressure, which may be uncomfortable.

If your doctor orders this test, you will be given advance instructions. The day before the procedure, you will be asked to drink a substance that cleanses the inside of your colon.

The double-contrast barium enema is not used as often as it once was. Although it is accurate enough to identify most large polyps and cancerous colorectal tumors, it can miss small polyps less than one inch in size.

Other Blood Tests

There is no specific blood test for colon cancer; however, your doctor may order blood tests if he or she suspects the presence of a colorectal cancer. A *complete blood count (CBC)* is a test performed to evaluate your red blood cell count. This test checks your hemoglobin and hematocrit. *Hemoglobin* is related to the amount of iron circulating in your blood. *Hematocrit* refers to the percentage of red blood cells in your total blood volume. If both values are lower than normal, you have a condition called *anemia.*

Anemia can be caused by slowly losing blood over several months from a growing colorectal cancer. However, having anemia does not necessarily mean you have colorectal cancer. Anemia can be caused by a number of other health problems.

A word of caution about blood tests: If you have an abnormal blood test, remember that abnormal test results alone do *not* necessarily mean you have colorectal cancer. Your doctor will need to put these results in perspective with your symptoms and the results of other tests before being able to determine whether cancer is present.

Other Diagnostic Tests

Your doctor may order other tests if he or she suspects colorectal cancer. Many times, these tests are ordered to evaluate whether a newly diagnosed cancer has spread to other parts of the body. The tests are also ordered in anticipation of treatment, such as surgery or chemotherapy. The tests are performed in an outpatient setting; they are noninvasive and involve no discomfort.

Computerized Axial Tomography (CAT) Scan

A *computerized axial tomography scan* is commonly referred to as a *CAT scan* or a *CT scan*. This type of scan uses special X-ray equipment and computers to take a series of detailed photos of the body's internal organs, tissues, bones, and blood vessels. If you have been diagnosed with colorectal cancer, the scan can help determine whether the cancer is confined to the colon or whether it may have spread.

For this test, you lie on an examination table that moves slowly through the scanning machine, which has a large hole in the middle of it. The machine takes pictures that are similar to X-rays; however, the images produced by the scan are much more detailed than standard X-rays.

Magnetic Resonance Imaging (MRI) Scan

The *magnetic resonance imagining (MRI) scan* is another type of scan that you may undergo. The scanning machine uses a combination of powerful magnets, radio frequency, and computers to take pictures of your soft tissues, bones, and other internal body structures. In some situations, an MRI is more effective in detecting abnormal tissues than other scans are. The MRI can also help determine whether a cancer has spread outside the colon or rectum.

For this test, you lie on an examination table that slides into a large, hollow tube. Because the MRI uses a powerful magnetic field, you cannot wear jewelry during the scan. Nor should you have any other metals with you, such as pens, watches, or eyeglasses, while undergoing the scan. People who should not have an MRI are those with metal screws, pins, or plates in their bodies; those with pacemakers; and those with cochlear ear implants. Also, if you are claustrophobic, talk to your doctor about taking a mild sedative prior to the test since you will spend fifteen to forty-five minutes inside the large cylinder. However, many testing centers now have "open MRIs," which you pass through without being confined to a cylinder.

Positron Emission Tomography (PET) Scan

The *positron emission tomography (PET) scan* provides internal photos that tell doctors how well organs and tissues are functioning; it allows them to observe such things as blood flow, oxygen use, and how the body uses glucose (sugar). This test is not typically used as an initial diagnostic tool, and when it is used, its usually used in combination with a CT scan. Doctors will often use a PET scan to help stage a cancer after surgery, when you're preparing for additional treatment such as chemotherapy.

For this test, you'll injected with a chemical that will move through your body; then, about an hour later, you'll lie on a table that will move through the scanner.

Ultrasound Test

Another diagnostic tool, an *ultrasound test* uses sound waves to produce pictures of internal organs. Ultrasound is often used to examine abdominal organs, specifically the liver, to check for any spread of colorectal cancer. The technician performing the test runs a device called a *transducer,* which resembles a microphone, over the body, and sound waves produce images on a video screen. *Transrectal ultrasound* involves placing a thin probe inside the rectum. If a tumor is present, the sound waves penetrate the tumor and provide information about how deeply the cancer has invaded the rectal wall or whether it has spread to lymph nodes. This information is important for surgical treatment.

X-rays

A standard X-ray is not used to diagnose colorectal cancer; however, it provides a physician with other information. For example, a chest X-ray can be used to check for any underlying lung disease or whether a cancer has spread to the lungs. A chest X-ray is usually ordered before surgery once a colorectal cancer is diagnosed. An X-ray of the abdomen can also determine whether a tumor might be blocking the intestines. X-rays can also be done to evaluate whether a newly diagnosed cancer has spread to the bones.

After the Diagnostic Tests

After your diagnostic tests, your physician will discuss the results with you. If you are diagnosed with colorectal cancer, you will be referred to other physicians who specialize in the treatment of cancer. Before treatment, however, the cancer will be staged, to estimate the extent to which it has penetrated tissues. Then, a treatment plan will be determined based on the stage of the cancer.

Coping Emotionally

As mentioned earlier, fear and anxiety are common reactions to the diagnosis of colorectal cancer. It's important to recognize and cope with such negative emotions because they can affect your health. Anxiety and stress can lead to lack of sleep, poor appetite, weight loss, and poor judgment. Research has shown that stress caused by negative emotions can depress the immune system and may impair recovery.

Getting emotional support from family and friends will help you cope. If you have loved ones who are not near by, you can stay in touch with them through several online sites. These Web sites, listed in the Resources section at the back of this book, allow you to create private pages where you can post updates about your hospital stays and treatments without making multiple phone calls or sending emails. You may also wish to consider contacting psychologists, counselors, ministers, or chaplains. Having good emotional support plays an important role in your journey through diagnosis and treatment.

Finding Support Services

Your healthcare team will likely have suggestions for you on where to find services for you and your family. Also, you can call the National Cancer Institute.

Information specialists will help you locate programs, services, and publications. You can speak with a specialist by calling 1-800-4-CANCER. Or, you can interact with a specialist online by going to "Live Help" at www.cancer.gov.

3 Staging Colorectal Cancer

The process of *staging* a newly discovered colorectal cancer involves determining the stage of the cancer's growth. For example, is the cancer at an early stage, meaning it has not spread beyond the colon or rectum? Or, has the cancer spread outside the colorectal wall, in which case it would be considered to be at a more advanced stage. Knowing the stage of a cancer is important because it helps doctors determine the treatment plan to follow.

There are two types of staging—clinical and pathological. The clinical stage is based on your doctor's clinical findings—diagnostic tests, including X-rays, scans, and biopsies—prior to any treatment. The pathological stage is based on clinical findings along with analysis of tissue and tumor samples after surgery, a common treatment for colorectal cancer. The staging based on the pathology report is the more accurate of the two types of staging, since tissue samples taken at the time of surgery may provide more-specific information about any spread of the cancer.

How Cancer Spreads
There are three ways cancer spreads. It can spread through surrounding tissue, through the lymph system, or through blood. It can spread through surrounding tissue by

first growing through the inner lining of the colon into the middle layer and ultimately through the outermost layer.

If the cancer extends through the entire colon wall, it can invade the adjacent *lymph nodes.* The lymph nodes are glands that filter the blood for infectious organisms as part of your immune system. There are hundreds of lymph nodes throughout your body. They are normally the size of a raisin when not inflamed or affected by cancer. You may notice that when you have a sore throat, the lymph nodes in your neck become enlarged because of the infection. In people with colorectal cancer, the lymph nodes adjacent to the tumor can be invaded by cancer cells.

Once cancer cells get into the lymph nodes, tumor cells can escape into the bloodstream and travel throughout the body. Beyond the lymph nodes, the liver is the most common site for cancer spread. This occurs because the blood supply from the entire colon drains into the liver first. Any tumor cells in the blood leaving the colon will first become lodged in the liver.

Colorectal cancer can also spread to the lungs, bones, bladder, brain, ovaries, and peritoneum (the thin lining surrounding all the abdominal organs). When a secondary tumor forms in any of these organs, these cancers are called *metastasis.*

Before your doctor can fully stage your colorectal cancer, he or she needs to answer the following questions:

- What is the extent of tumor growth through the colon wall?
- Are the lymph nodes near the cancer involved with the tumor?
- Has the cancer spread to other organs?

The answers to the first two questions can only be obtained after you undergo surgery and the cancerous tissue and lymph nodes are removed.

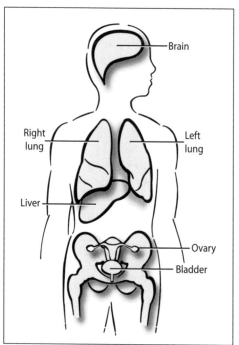

Areas to which colorectal cancer can spread include the brain, lungs, liver, ovaries, and bladder.

Pathology Report

After surgery, a *pathologist*, a doctor who examines tissues and organs for diseases, will perform laboratory tests on the tissue removed. Once testing of the tissue specimens is complete, he or she will deliver a written pathology report. This report will tell your physician whether the cancer has spread through the colorectal wall and whether lymph nodes are involved. It usually takes two to four days after surgery to obtain a final pathology report. The pathology report will determine your cancer stage, taking into consideration the factors listed below.

Type of Cancer Cells Present

Once the abnormal tissue is studied by the pathologist, the type of cancer cells present can be determined. The types include benign, precancerous, noninvasive, and invasive. As mentioned earlier, "benign" means noncancerous. "Precancerous" means the growth has the potential to become cancer. "Noninvasive" means the cancer is limited to the lining of the colon. "Invasive" cancers are those that have invaded into or beyond the wall of the colon.

Degree of Differentiation

The degree of differentiation refers to how much the cancer cells resemble the normal cells. There are three degrees of differentiation: poorly, moderately, and well differentiated. Poorly differentiated cancer cells are chaotic, more aggressive than the other two types, and have the worst prognosis. Well-differentiated cancer cells are not as aggressive and have the best prognosis.

Spread to Blood Vessels

Known as *extramural venous invasion*, this condition means the cancer cells have invaded the walls of the small blood vessels surrounding the tumor and have the potential to leak into the bloodstream. This is not a favorable characteristic, as it increases the risk of spread to other organs in the body.

Resection Margins

The term "resection" refers to the surgical removal of a cancer. The *resection margins* refer to the tissue in the margins, or around the edges, of the tumor. The pathologist will analyze these tissues for evidence of cancer cells. If the resection margins are free of cancer cells, it's an indication that all the cancerous tissue was removed during the surgery. But if the resection margins contain cancer cells, further treatment will be required.

Extent of Tumor Growth

This part of the report describes how far the cancer has grown into the colorectal wall. The best-case scenario has the tumor confined to the inner layer. The worst-case scenario has the tumor growing through all the layers and invading the *pericolonic fat*. In such a case, the chances are high for *recurrence* of the cancer. In addition, the further a cancer grows through the colorectal wall, the greater the chance of it spreading to the lymph nodes.

Lymph Node Involvement

The report will tell whether cancer has invaded any lymph nodes. If the lymph nodes are negative, it means no cancerous cells were found in the lymph nodes. According to today's standard of care, if at least twelve lymph nodes are negative, the surgery is considered successful in removing all the cancer.

A report of positive lymph nodes means cancer cells are present and further treatment will be needed. In addition, the number of lymph nodes involved is a factor in determining prognosis.

Stage I: The cancer has not spread to the colon wall.

Stage II: The cancer has spread to the middle layers of the colon wall.

Stages of Colon Cancer

Taking all the information from the pathology report, doctors will classify the stage of your cancer. The stages range from 0 to IV.

Stage 0: In stage 0, abnormal cells are found in the innermost lining of the colon. These abnormal cells may become cancer and spread into nearby normal tissue. This stage is also called carcinoma in situ.

Stage I: Cancer has formed and spread beyond the innermost tissue layer of the colon wall to the middle layers.

Stage II: In stage II, colon cancer is divided into stages IIA and IIB.

Stage IIA: Cancer has spread beyond the middle tissue layers of the colon wall or has spread to nearby tissues around the colon or rectum.

Stage IIB: Cancer has spread beyond the colon wall into

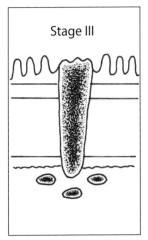

Stage III: the cancer has spread to nearby tissues and lymph nodes.

Stage IV: the cancer has spread to other organs such as the liver and lung.

nearby organs and/or through the peritoneum.

Stage III: In stage III, colon cancer is divided into stage IIIA, stage IIIB, and stage IIIC.

Stage IIIA: Cancer has spread from the innermost tissue layer of the colon wall to the middle layers and has spread to as many as three lymph nodes.

Stage IIIB: Cancer has spread to as many as three nearby

lymph nodes and has spread beyond the middle tissue layers of the colon wall, or to nearby tissues around the colon or rectum, or beyond the colon wall into nearby organs and/or through the peritoneum.

Stage IIIC: Cancer has spread to four or more nearby lymph nodes and has spread to or beyond the middle tissue layers of the colon wall, or to nearby tissues around the colon or rectum, or to nearby organs and/or through the peritoneum.

Stage IV: Cancer may have spread to nearby lymph nodes and has spread to other parts of the body, such as the liver or lungs.

Stages of Rectal Cancer

Stage 0: In stage 0, abnormal cells are found in the innermost lining of the rectum. These abnormal cells may become cancer and spread into nearby normal tissue. Stage 0 is also called carcinoma in situ.

Stage I: In stage I, cancer has formed and spread beyond the innermost lining of the rectum to the second and third layers and involves the inside wall of the rectum, but it has not spread to the outer wall of the rectum or outside the rectum.

Stage II: In stage II, cancer has spread outside the rectum to nearby tissue, but it has not gone into the lymph nodes.

Stage III: In stage III, cancer has spread to nearby lymph nodes, but it has not spread to other parts of the body.

Stage IV: In stage IV, cancer has spread to other parts of the body, such as the liver, lungs, or ovaries.

Note: If you wish to learn more specific information about the system doctors use for classifying the extent to which a cancer has spread, see the "TNM Classification System" in the Appendix.

Treatment Planning

As soon as the stage of a cancer is determined, doctors can recommend the best type of treatment. For an early-stage colon or rectal cancer, treatment may involve surgery alone; in some cases chemotherapy or radiation may also be recommended. For other stages of colon or rectal cancer, most treatment plans involve surgery along with chemotherapy or radiation or a combination of both chemotherapy and radiation.

In the chapters that follow, you'll read about each of these treatment options.

4 Surgery

If the colorectal cancer has not spread to other organs, the first line of treatment is surgery. For most newly diagnosed colorectal cancer patients, surgery is the primary treatment and offers the best chance for a cure. The goal of any operation for colorectal cancer is to remove the portion of the colon or rectum that contains the growing cancer, along with the surrounding lymph nodes.

Colorectal surgery is performed by general surgeons and colorectal surgeons. These physicians may perform one of several different types of surgery, depending on the location and stage of your cancer.

Surgeries for Colon Cancer

Polypectomy

The surgery to remove a polyp is called a *polypectomy*. A polypectomy is often performed by a gastroenterologist or surgeon during a colonoscopy. In this procedure, the doctor uses an assortment of wires, snares, and small forceps to remove a polyp through the colonoscope while you are sedated. The procedure is usually done on an outpatient basis.

Most polyps that are under one inch in diameter and growing on a stalk, like a mushroom, can be removed this way. However, polyps larger than one inch in diameter, broad based, or containing cancer cells require an operation to remove a part of the colon and the surrounding lymph nodes.

Open Partial Colectomy

The most common type of surgery for colon cancer, an *open partial colectomy* is the removal of part of the colon. The term "open" refers to the fact that an incision is made and the abdomen is "opened." This is major surgery and requires anesthesia. During the operation, the surgeon makes a six- to twelve-inch vertical incision in the middle of your abdomen and removes the segment of the colon that is cancerous.

The type of partial colectomy you may need depends on where the tumor is located. If the cancer is located in the right colon, the operation performed is called a *right colectomy* since only the right part of the colon is removed. To remove a cancer in the transverse colon, a *transverse colectomy* is needed. A cancer located in the left colon is removed by a *left colectomy*. One located in the sigmoid colon is removed by a *sigmoid colectomy*.

When performing a partial colectomy, surgeons want to have at least six inches of normal colon tissue surrounding either side of the segment that is removed. The six inches of normal colon tissue is called the margin. An adequate margin of normal colon tissue minimizes the risk of the cancer coming back in the same area after the two ends are reconnected.

After the cancerous section of the colon is removed, the surgeon reattaches the two ends of the colon. They are joined together by either sutures or metal staples. If sutures are used, your body will absorb them over several months. If metal staples are used, they are left in place permanently. Both techniques are equally effective.

The surgery takes from one to three hours and commonly involves a five- to seven-day recovery in the hospital.

Surgeries for Colorectal Cancer

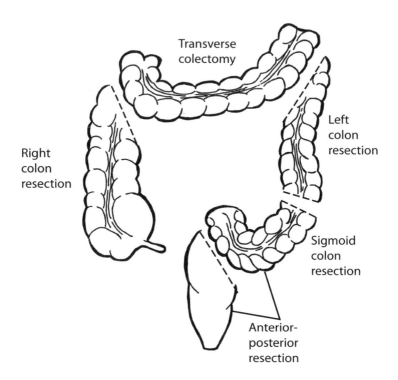

Open Subtotal and Total Colectomies

An *open subtotal colectomy* is a surgical procedure in which more than 90 percent of the colon is removed. It's not a common operation; however, it may be necessary when a person has two separate colon cancers in two different parts of the colon. During this major abdominal operation, the surgeon is still able to reattach both ends of normal colon once the two cancerous segments are removed.

An *open total colectomy* removes the entire colon. Again, this is not a common operation for colon cancer. It is generally performed for other diseases of the colon.

Both of these operations take about three hours and involve a seven-day recovery in the hospital.

Surgeries for Rectal Cancer

Polypectomy

A rectal polyp can also be removed through the colonoscope at the time of a colonoscopy. Most polyps found in the rectum can be removed this way. However, rectal polyps greater than one inch in diameter and with a broad base may be difficult to remove without an operation. In addition, polyps found to have cancer in them once removed by the colonoscope may require more-extensive surgery.

Transanal Excision

The *transanal excision* of a polyp or early cancer in the rectum involves surgical removal through the anus. This is a unique approach since most operations for colorectal cancer involve making a six- to twelve-inch vertical incision through the middle of the abdomen. By operating through the anus and not the abdominal cavity, there is much less trauma to the body and less physical pain. This approach is appropriate if you have a polyp just inside the anus that is not cancerous and cannot be removed at the time of colonoscopy.

The transanal approach might also be appropriate, and can save you from undergoing a much larger operation, if you have a small polyp with some early cancerous cells present just inside the anus. However, additional treatment such as radiation may be needed to kill any potential cancer cells left behind.

The operation is carried out under general anesthesia and takes about one hour. It can be performed in an outpatient setting or in a hospital. Some patients may need to stay overnight in the hospital.

Open Low Anterior Resection

An *open low anterior resection* removes a cancer located in the lower one-third of the sigmoid colon or upper two-thirds of the rectum. This major operation is very effective. It involves general anesthesia and takes approximately two hours. During the procedure, the surgeon makes a vertical incision starting above the belly button and removes about a twelve-inch portion of the sigmoid colon and rectum. The adjacent lymph nodes are also removed. After removing the cancerous segment, the surgeon reattaches the two free ends together so normal bowel movements can occur. Recovery in the hospital takes at least seven days.

Open Anterior-Posterior Resection

An *open anterior-posterior resection,* or *AP resection,* is performed on rectal cancers located just inside the anus. The operation takes three hours, requires general anesthesia, and involves a twelve-inch vertical incision in your abdomen. When a cancer is located less than six to twelve inches from the outside of the anus, this operation may offer the best chance for a cure. If the surgeon can feel the cancer during a rectal examination, then chances are an anterior-posterior resection is the necessary operation.

The procedure involves removing the cancerous section of the rectum and the anus. When the anus is removed, it is no longer possible to have normal bowel movements. So, during the surgery, the surgeon will perform a *colostomy,* a procedure that connects the colon to an opening on the surface of the lower abdomen. An external colostomy bag is attached to the new opening. Now, fecal matter will no longer pass through the anus, but will pass into this bag. You'll learn more about colostomies at the end of this chapter.

Pelvic Exenteration

A *pelvic exenteration* is to be considered when a cancer of the rectum has invaded nearby organs, such as the bladder, uterus, or ovaries. In this situation, the best chance for curing a patient is to remove all the organs attached to the rectal cancer at once, without disturbing any cancer cells. This major operation is seldom performed today.

Minimally Invasive Surgery

Also known as *laparoscopic surgery*, a *minimally invasive surgery* is performed more frequently today to treat a variety of diseases, including colorectal cancer. Unlike open surgeries, in which large incisions are made, these procedures involve making small incisions in the abdomen. Thin, fiber-optic cameras attached to television monitors are then inserted and become the "eyes" of the surgeons as they manipulate their instruments. Smaller incisions mean less pain after surgery, quicker recovery in the hospital, fewer scars, and a shorter time needed to get back to a normal routine.

Minimally invasive surgery for colorectal cancer is available in many cities. However, these operations are complex and are more difficult for surgeons to master than the traditional operations involving larger incisions. Many surgeons are not experienced in this approach and do not perform minimally invasive surgery.

Undergoing Major Surgery

Once you are in the operating room, an *anesthesiologist* will inject medication into your IV to put you to sleep. Within seconds, this general anesthesia will take effect, and you will be unconscious and won't be able to feel or hear anything. A *nasogastric tube*, placed down your throat and into your stomach, will suction out any accumulation of fluid, that could cause vomiting.

Surgery for colon cancer is major surgery. The most common procedure involves removal of a portion of the colon.

During the operation, your surgeon will remove the cancerous segment of your colon and reconnect the two free ends together. Your surgeon will also visually inspect all the other organs in your abdominal cavity to look for evidence that the cancer has spread. If a suspicious nodule or mass is found, especially in the liver, the surgeon will remove a piece of tissue for laboratory examination (biopsy). Once the operation is complete, the breathing tube is removed before you wake up; however, the surgeon may leave the nasogastric tube in place so it can continue to suction any fluid buildup over the next two to four days. Once the anesthesiologist gives the okay, you will be placed back on a gurney and taken to the recovery room.

In the recovery room, your vital signs (blood pressure, heart rate, and respiration rate) will be closely monitored and checked by the nurses. When your surgeon determines that you are stable, you'll be moved to a hospital room.

Recovery in the Hospital

Barring any major complications, most patients need a week in the hospital to recover from major colorectal cancer surgery. Complications may keep you in the hospital longer. The physical stress from the operation typically interrupts normal body functions, and it may take a few days for these functions to return to normal. During this time, your surgeon will see you every day. He or she will monitor your recovery and decide when to remove tubes, when to decrease your pain medicine, when to have your dressing changed, when you should get out of bed, and when you should be fed. All these decisions are dependent upon how soon your bodily functions return to normal.

Pain Management after Surgery

Prior to surgery, be sure to discuss ways to manage your postoperative pain with your surgeon. Don't wait until you're groggy after surgery to discuss this important issue.

There are several methods for controlling pain. You can be given periodic injections of narcotic drugs. You can be hooked up to a *patient-controlled anesthesia (PCA)* pump that administers a continuous dose of narcotics over a twenty-four-hour period. The PCA pump also allows you to administer additional narcotic booster injections through a handheld device if the pain worsens. The PCA pump provides steadier, more even postoperative pain control than traditional injections.

An *epidural* catheter is another form of pain management. The catheter is a tiny, soft plastic tube that an anesthesiologist inserts in the middle of your back and guides close to your spinal cord. The medication affects the nerves that cause you to feel pain from the surgery. The catheter may be left in place for several days after surgery. It is an effective way to control pain after major abdominal operations.

Once you begin to drink liquids or eat solid food, your surgeon will likely switch from intravenous pain medications to oral medications. These should be taken as directed, to stay ahead of the pain. Don't wait until you're in pain to take the medications.

Your postoperative pain should lessen with each passing day. If your pain is not being adequately controlled, tell your nurse or your surgeon. Tolerating pain should not be part of the normal healing process. You are not being a bothersome patient by asking for help with pain relief.

Regaining Bowel Function

You'll need to regain normal bowel function before you can be released from the hospital. Any major abdominal surgery on either the small or large intestine causes the intestines to "go to sleep." Your surgeon's handling of the small intestine or colon during the process of removing a segment traumatizes the intestines and causes them to temporarily stop working. This is called *postoperative ileus* ("ileus" means "slowing down"). It is a normal response to major abdominal surgery. Postoperative ileus lasts three to five days and is completely reversible.

During this period, your intestines will not be able to move liquid waste products toward the anus for removal, so fluid can back up into the stomach. This backup can cause you to feel nauseous and result in vomiting. Food given to you during this time will make you feel sick. The nasogastric tube will continue to suction fluid buildup. When your health-care team begins to hear bowel sounds—growling noises in your abdomen—it is a sign that your intestines are becoming active. When this occurs, your surgeon will likely remove the nasogastric tube. You will likely be able to start drinking liquids to see if your stomach can tolerate them. If so, regular food will soon follow.

During this time, you may begin to pass gas and may experience loose bowel movements that come on very suddenly. You may also pass a small amount of blood with initial bowel movements. Both gas and a little bleeding are normal.

Note that if you undergo a minimally invasive surgery, the intestines are "inactive" for a shorter period of time, and often, the surgeon will remove the nasogastric tube at the end of the operation.

Keeping the Lungs Expanded

After the operation, the nurses caring for you will tell you to practice deep breathing and coughing. Placing a pillow on your stomach and holding it as you cough will also ease the pain immediately after surgery. Deep breaths help keep the lungs expanded to prevent pneumonia. If you smoke or have a history of lung disease, deep breathing is especially important.

Because deep breathing hurts after major abdominal surgery, it is natural to want to take short, incomplete breaths. Concentrate on your breathing while recovering in the hospital. An *incentive spirometer* can help you keep your lungs expanded. This is a tubelike device you breathe through that has a gauge that shows how well your lungs expand by measuring how deep your breathing is.

Blowing into an incentive spirometer helps keep the lungs expanded after surgery. *Photo by CMSP*

Blood Tests

For several days after your operation, blood will be taken from your arm each morning to evaluate your blood count. Since these lab values will fluctuate after major abdominal surgery, your surgeon needs to monitor them during recovery.

If your blood count drops too low, you may require a transfusion. A low blood count can lead to low blood pressure, fatigue, and potentially a heart attack if you have a history of heart problems. Other abnormalities in the blood can lead to abnormal heart rhythms and seizures and can prolong the inactivity of the intestines following surgery.

Regaining Mobility

Getting out of bed and walking in your room or in the hallway as soon as you are physically able is also important for a fast, uncomplicated recovery. Walking gets the blood circulating, prevents blood clots from forming, and may help you regain intestinal function more quickly. Walking, like coughing and deep breathing, will cause some initial discomfort. However, as each day passes, it will become easier. Walking may be difficult while you're connected to tubes and intravenous lines. The nurses or a therapist will assist you.

Planning for Additional Treatment

Before discharge, your surgeon will talk to you about your pathology report and whether further treatment is needed. If so, your surgeon will call an *oncologist* for consultation. An oncologist is a doctor trained in the medical treatment of cancer.

Discharge from the Hospital

As your hospital stay draws to an end, you should be walking as much as possible and eating normal food. Your bowel movements should be close to normal, and the pain from your incision should be adequately controlled with oral pain medication.

On the day you're discharged from the hospital, you will be given instructions for managing postoperative pain; usually, you will be given a prescription for painkillers. You'll also be given guidelines for levels of activity that are appropriate for you, along with instructions for such activities as bathing.

If your surgeon used metal staples to close your incision, they will need to be removed during a follow-up office appointment, usually in seven to ten days. (These staples are different from those used internally to connect the segments of your colon.)

Possible Complications of Colorectal Surgery

The risk for complications after colorectal cancer surgery depends on a number of factors. Your overall health and any preexisting medical conditions can affect whether you develop complications. If you have high blood pressure, a heart condition, lung disease, or diabetes, you are at a slightly higher risk for developing complications. People who have diabetes and/or who are obese, for instance, are prone to develop wound infections after surgery. Your risk for complications is minimal if you are healthy, do not smoke, are physically active, and are not overweight.

Whether your surgery is planned or performed on an emergency basis also impacts your risk for complications. A planned operation takes place in a controlled setting under optimum conditions so the risks are small. Emergency surgery has a higher complication rate.

Complications following colorectal surgery are relatively rare, occurring in less than 5 percent of patients. However, the complications can be life threatening if they aren't recognized and treated immediately. Possible complications include heart attack, pneumonia, wound infection, blood clots in the legs (with potential spread to the lungs, causing death), intra-abdominal infection or associated abscess, and *fistula*. A fistula is an abnormal connection between the intestine and the skin. A fistula occurs when the intestine is punctured and stool leaks out. It can lead to a serious infection requiring antibiotics. Most fistulas, however, heal spontaneously and do not require surgery.

Even in the 5 percent of patients who do experience

postsurgical complications, most respond to treatment and do not require further surgery.

Recovery at Home

Recovering at home after colorectal cancer surgery can take four to eight weeks. While at home, it is normal to initially not have much of an appetite. Most people lose ten to twenty pounds following surgery. Your appetite will improve over the next several weeks. Most often, you'll be free to eat whatever you'd like.

Watch for any signs of infection—fever, any drainage, redness, increasing pain from your abdominal incision, and coughing up dark sputum. All these are warning signs of infection, and your surgeon needs to be notified immediately. Your bowel habits should quickly return to normal once you return home. Persistent diarrhea while at home is *not* normal. Let your surgeon know if this occurs. Persistent nausea, abdominal pain, and vomiting are also not normal and also should be reported.

Do not expect to have a normal energy level right away. It will take one to two months for your energy to return to the preoperative level. Do not try to do too much too fast. Limit your activities, and do not expect to return to work for at least one month. Expect your energy level to fluctuate, alternating between good days and bad days. This is completely normal after major colorectal surgery.

In addition to being a physical strain, recovering at home from colorectal cancer surgery can be full of emotional ups and downs. This kind of mental stress is especially prevalent when you are at home, inactive, and recovering, with plenty of time to think. Try to keep busy at home with hobbies and things that exercise your mental capabilities.

Do not be afraid to open up to family and friends. Talk with them about how you're feeling, your fears, and your concerns. Try to maintain a positive outlook. Some people find comfort in cancer support groups; such groups can provide moral support and practical advice for recovery. Also, consider talking with friends, neighbors, and coworkers who have had cancer and have gone through treatment.

If You Need a Colostomy

As mentioned earlier, colostomy refers to the creation of an opening in the lower abdomen after the anus has been removed. A colostomy bag, attached to the opening, collects waste.

According to the National Cancer Institute, about 15 percent of people who undergo surgery for colorectal cancer require a permanent colostomy. Whether or not you need a colostomy depends on the size and location of the tumor. After this has been determined by the diagnostic tests, your surgeon will talk with you about the specifics of such a procedure.

Temporary Colostomy

Sometimes, a temporary colostomy is required after emergency colon surgery. In these cases, a colostomy helps avoid serious infections. For example, you may need emergency surgery to have a blockage in your colon removed. Or, you may need emergency surgery if cancer has perforated the colon wall, causing feces and bacteria to spill into the abdomen. Since there is no time to cleanse the colon prior to surgery, the risk of infection is high if two ends of a "dirty" colon are sewn together after a cancerous segment has been removed. The best way to minimize this risk is to perform a temporary colostomy at the time of the operation.

A temporary colostomy usually remains in place for four to six months, enough time for healing after the surgery. Then, in another operation, the surgeon can go back and reconnect the colon sections. This reversal of the colostomy is called a *colostomy takedown*. It is a major operation that takes several hours and involves general anesthesia and a week's recovery in the hospital. Colostomy takedown restores normal bowel function.

Permanent Colostomy

A permanent colostomy is required if the cancer is located in the rectum close to the anus and the surgeon must remove the entire rectum and part of the colon. In this case, it is no longer possible to reattach the colon to the rectum. As a result, a colostomy is needed.

If you have a colostomy, its location on your abdomen will usually be determined before surgery. For most individuals, the colostomy is located below and to the left of the navel. It is uncommon to find colostomies located elsewhere in the abdomen.

Wearing a Colostomy Bag

To attach the colostomy bag, first a plastic adhesive barrier, shaped like a doughnut, is placed around the opening in the abdomen. This opening is called a stoma. Then, the external plastic pouch is attached to the adhesive barrier. The pouch fits under your clothes and is usually not noticeable to others.

Colostomy Care

While you're in the hospital, you may see an *enterostomal nurse*, a registered nurse specially trained in the care of colostomies. In addition to explaining how to care for your colostomy, this nurse will provide other information such as where to get supplies in your community.

Caring for your colostomy at home is not difficult. The pouch needs to be emptied into the toilet periodically during the day as it fills up. You can empty the pouch by opening a plastic clip at its base and allowing the fecal material to spill into the toilet. After the pouch has been emptied, the plastic clip can be reattached and the bottom of the pouch closed. Most people become very adept at emptying the pouch and do not have problems with soiled garments or lingering odors. Drops of deodorizer can be dropped into the bag immediately after it is emptied. There are several specialized liquid deodorizers that may be purchased at medical supply stores.

Colostomy Bag

Irrigating your colostomy with a simple saline solution will be helpful if it becomes clogged. Essentially, colostomy irrigation works like an enema. Ask your nurse or doctor about irrigation and how to do it. The plastic pouch itself usually needs to be replaced every five to seven days. The colostomy opening may be washed with soap and water.

When it's necessary for the surgeon to remove the anus, an external colostomy bag is needed to collect waste. About 15 percent of people with colorectal cancer require a colostomy.

Most people with colostomies keep extra supplies nearby just in case they are needed unexpectedly. Make sure you have plenty of supplies at home. Colostomy supplies can be obtained in some drugstores and in many medical supply stores.

You do *not* need to be on a special diet with a colostomy. However, certain foods can affect the consistency of your colostomy output. Some foods may cause diarrhea or excess gas. Other foods may cause constipation. You can exert some control over your colostomy bowel habits by modifying your diet. By watching what you eat and eating at regular intervals, you can control when your colostomy works during the day. Ask your doctor about how foods affect your colostomy; your doctor may help you with this or may refer you to a dietician.

Emotional Support

At first, accepting the fact that you have a colostomy may be emotionally difficult. You may experience feelings of depression, frustration, anger, sadness, and isolation. You may withdraw from family and friends. It's important to realize that all these feelings and reactions are common. Talk with those you trust—your physician, family members, and friends. Consider seeking out cancer and colostomy support groups in your area. They can provide valuable insights and help you cope with your new situation.

Colostomy's Effect on Sexual Activity

Many people wonder if a colostomy will affect their sex lives. Usually, individuals who have colostomies can have active sex lives. Women normally have no loss of sexual function due to colostomy. However, some men who have had colostomies do not ejaculate, or they may have a retrograde emission, in which semen is forced backward into the bladder. This may occur because tiny nerves located deep in the pelvis, near the rectum, may be damaged during surgery. Surgeons try to avoid damaging these nerves, but if damage occurs, the emission of semen may be affected. A man's ability to attain an erection is not changed, but pleasurable sensations during sexual activity may be slightly diminished. Still, with a few changes, most individuals adapt and continue having a normal sex life.

Potential Complications

Most people do not have complications with their colostomy. However, one of the most common problems that occurs is the development of a hernia around the stoma. Symptoms of a hernia include a bulge in the skin around the stoma, problems with irrigating, or blockages. Seek medical attention if you experience any of the following symptoms:

- Severe cramps that last for more than two to three hours

- Watery discharge from the stoma for more than six hours
- No output from the colostomy for several days
- unusual odor that lasts more than a week
- Bleeding from the stoma or seeing blood in the pouch
- Stoma pulling inward or narrowing
- Chronic skin irritation

Another possible problem is rubbing or irritation from the pouch that may cause skin abrasions; your physician may prescribe topical ointments.

Life after Receiving a Colostomy

People with colostomies live normal, active lives. A colostomy does not mean your lifestyle needs to change dramatically. Initially, a colostomy presents physical and emotional challenges. However, with the proper education and support, these challenges can be overcome. After you've recovered from your operation, you can exercise, wear normal clothes, and return to work without feeling awkward or embarrassed.

5 Chemotherapy

Chemotherapy plays a major role in cancer treatment. It is used to help cure, control, or ease the symptoms of cancer. Nearly half of all cancer patients undergo chemotherapy.

To explain how chemotherapy works, first keep in mind that all cells in our bodies go through growth cycles—cells reproduce and then they rest. Some normal cells grow rapidly, while other normal cells reproduce more slowly. Cancer cells divide rapidly, and chemotherapy destroys only cells that are reproducing rapidly. It can also damage healthy cells, but those cells are capable of recovering.

If your doctors decide chemotherapy is right for you, you'll meet with a medical oncologist, a doctor that specializes in chemotherapy. He or she will formulate a chemotherapy plan to treat your cancer.

Chemotherapy after Surgery

When chemotherapy is given *after* surgery, it is called *adjuvant chemotherapy.* It is used with the intention of killing any cancer cells that might remain after surgery. For colorectal cancer, adjuvant chemotherapy is given when the cancer has spread through the wall of the colon or rectum or has entered the lymph nodes. Other factors that determine whether chemotherapy is appropriate include the type of cancer, how aggressive it is, the patient's age, and the overall health of the patient.

If you've undergone surgery, your physician will probably wait three to four weeks before beginning chemotherapy, allowing you to heal.

Most chemotherapy treatments for colon cancer after surgery continue for six months, with a treatment every two weeks.

Chemotherapy before Surgery

When chemotherapy is given *before* surgery, it is known as *neoadjuvant chemotherapy.* Chemotherapy prior to surgery is given in an effort to shrink a cancer so that the chances are increased for removing the entire tumor and killing cancer cells that may have traveled to other parts of the body.

Neoadjuvant chemotherapy is not typically used for colon cancer, because surgery is considered an effective first-line treatment. However, neoadjuvant chemotherapy is sometimes recommended for rectal cancer; this is done for two reasons— in an attempt to preserve the anal sphincter and to reduce the chances for recurrence in the rectum. When cancers are found near the anus, it is often impossible to preserve the anal sphincter with surgery alone; however, when chemotherapy is given prior to the surgery, the sphincter can be saved more than 50 percent of the time. If the sphincter is removed, the patient requires a colostomy, an opening in the abdomen for collecting waste.

Chemotherapy before rectal cancer surgery usually lasts four to six weeks, with surgery following three to four weeks later. The chemotherapy may also be recommended *after* the surgery for rectal cancer; in this case, the chemotherapy usually continues for four to six months.

Palliative Chemotherapy

Another form of treatment, palliative chemotherapy is given to provide relief from symptoms. Palliative chemotherapy may be an option when cancer has already spread to other organs, such as the liver, lungs, or bones, at the time of initial diagnosis or at the time of surgery and is considered incurable. In such cases, chemotherapy may shrink the tumor and slow its growth.

Receiving Chemotherapy Treatments

Chemotherapy treatments are given in cycles—usually every two weeks. You receive a treatment, followed by a two-week recovery period. Then, you'll have another treatment, followed by another recovery period. Why are treatments given in cycles? As explained earlier, chemotherapy kills the cancer cells that are rapidly dividing; however, it won't affect those cells that are at rest. By making the treatments ongoing, the effort is intensified to kill cancer cells when they are in the reproduction phase. The time off between treatments also helps normal tissues recover.

Most chemotherapy treatments are given intravenously—treatments are called infusions. Indeed, pills would be easier, but stomach acids and enzymes would break down some medications and prevent them from working. (There is one chemotherapy drug, Capecitabine, that is given in pill form.)

Treatments are given in an outpatient setting, usually in a hospital's infusion center or at another outpatient site. A nurse who specializes in giving chemotherapy treatments will connect the intravenous line that delivers the chemotherapy. Before the treatment, patients are first given anti-nausea medication. Nurses monitor patients carefully during treatments.

While you're receiving an infusion, you'll usually be seated in a comfortable reclining chair; the treatment may last from one and one-half hours to four hours, depending on the chemotherapy agents used. During this time, you'll be able to read, watch television, use a laptop computer, or have visitors.

Chemotherapy through a Port

Chemotherapy for colorectal cancer is given over an extended period of time. So, to make the treatment process more efficient and more comfortable for you, your doctor will want to avoid your receiving a new IV line in your arm during each treatment. Accordingly, your chemotherapy may be delivered through a *port*.

A port is a small reservoir, about the size of a quarter often made of soft plastic. This port is surgically implanted in your chest just under the skin—usually under the collarbone. A soft, thin tube runs from the port into a large vein. The implantation of the port is an outpatient procedure, performed by your surgeon, and takes thirty to sixty minutes. Local anesthesia is used, and you may be given a mild sedative. After the procedure, a chest X-ray is done to check the positioning of the port and to make sure there is no kink in the tube. From this point, you'll receive your infusions through this port. When not in use, the port is covered with a bandage; once the small incision heals, no bandage is needed. The port requires no special care by the patient.

Ports rarely create complications; however, pain, redness, or swelling may indicate infection or clotting. You should report any such symptoms to your doctor immediately. Once you have completed your treatments, your surgeon will remove the port during an office visit.

Port

Before chemotherapy begins, a surgeon may implant a port, a small reservoir, under the skin. Chemotherapy infusions will be given through this port.

Chemotherapy through a Pump

When you are receiving an infusion at a treatment center, your chemotherapy drug may flow from a pump, which hangs from a pole. A needle that is attached to a soft, plastic tube leading from the pump is inserted into your port.

After you've finished such treatment, your oncologist may want you to continue receiving the chemotherapy drug for a number of days. You will be asked to wear an *ambulatory infusion pump*, a lightweight, battery-operated pump that attaches to a waist belt. This pump releases the chemotherapy drug into the bloodstream at a slow, even rate. Some colorectal

cancer patients may receive their drugs through the pump for several days at a time before taking a break. The pump is portable, and you'll wear it around the clock, even while you sleep.

Monitoring during Treatment

You'll be monitored closely while you're undergoing chemotherapy. Your blood count will be taken to measure your red blood cells, platelets, and white blood cells. Your doctor will be watching for blood counts that drop too low; for example, if your white blood cell count drops, you'll be at risk for infections since white blood cells fight infections.

Chemotherapy treatments are often delivered through an ambulatory infusion pump, which attaches to a belt. The pump will deliver chemotherapy while you're at home. *Photo courtesy of Outpatient Infusion Systems*

In most people, blood counts drop to their lowest levels seven to ten days after each treatment. This lowest point is called the *nadir*. When you are at your nadir, your immune system is weakened, and you will be susceptible to viruses and infections. You may require medications that boost your white blood cell count during this period.

Chemotherapy Agents

The medications used for chemotherapy consist of a group of different drugs, just as the term "antibiotics" refers to many different types of medications. Chemotherapy medications may be used alone, or they may be combined with each other.

Some chemotherapy drugs work by attacking the cancer cells' DNA, which is a cell's "blueprint" for growing and reproducing; these drugs interrupt the cells' ability to reproduce. Other chemotherapy drugs work by attacking cell molecules, such as those involved with blood-vessel formation.

Side Effects of Chemotherapy

Chemotherapy used to treat colorectal cancer is generally well tolerated by most people. As mentioned earlier, chemotherapy kills cancer cells that are rapidly reproducing. However, chemotherapy drugs will also attack the normal, healthy cells that reproduce rapidly. As a result, side effects occur.

The type of chemotherapy you receive, the dosage, and the duration of your treatment are factors in the types of side effects you may experience. It's important to note that not all patients experience every side effect, and when side effects do occur, they can usually be managed with prescription medications or even home remedies. Most side effects subside once the treatments end. A list of potential side effects follows.

Diarrhea

One of the most common side effects of chemotherapy used to treat colorectal cancer is diarrhea. It is caused by

Chemotherapy Agents for Colorectal Cancer	
Fluorouracil (5-FU)	This drug is commonly given as a three- to five-minute infusion at a treatment center; then, most patients will also receive the drug coninuously over one to four days through a small infusion pump worn at home. This treatment may be repeated weekly, every other week, or every three weeks. Flourouracil is used incombination with other chemotherapy drugs.
Capecitabine (Xeloda)	This agent, used alone, is taken as a daily pill, thirty minutes after a meal. It is often taken in divided dosages, twelve hours apart. Many oncologists recommend taking the pill for fourteen days in a row, then taking a seven-day break. The cycle is then repeated.
Oxaliplatin (Eloxatin)	Given by infusion intravenously over a two-hour period, this drug is usually given every two weeks. It is combined with other chemotherapy agents and a vitamin-like drug called leucovorin.
Irinotecan (Camptosar)	This agent is given intravenously over ninety minutes or longer when it is combined with other agents. Typically, it is given once every three weeks or weekly for four weeks.
Bevacizumab (Avastin)	This drug is given intravenously over ninety minutes; however, infusion time may gradually be reduced to thirty minutes if the drug is well tolerated. It may be combined with other chemotherapy drugs. Treatments are typically scheduled for every two weeks.
Cetuximab (Erbitux)	This drug is usually infused over a two-hour period, once a week. It may be used alone or in combination with other agents.
Panitumumab (Vectibix)	Used alone, this drug is given by intravenous infusion over sixty to ninety minutes; it is usually given every two weeks.

This man is receiving a chemotherapy infusion at an outpatient treatment center. Treatments are typically given in cycles—every two weeks. *Photo by PHOTOTAKE*

chemotherapy acting on the lining on the inside of the stomach and intestines. Abdominal cramping can also accompany diarrhea. Both may last several hours to several days. The concern about diarrhea is that, if not treated, it can lead to dehydration. If diarrhea becomes severe, you may need to have fluids replaced intravenously; hospitalization may be required.

Since diarrhea can cause the body to lose a large amount of water in a short period of time, you can also lose important minerals and *electrolytes*. If you're having diarrhea, take these measures:

- Drink at least six to eight glasses of water daily.
- Avoid high-fiber, greasy, and spicy foods.
- Eat small amounts of solid food frequently throughout the day.

What Is KRAS Testing?

KRAS testing involves the testing of tumor tissue after surgery, helping oncologists determine which chemotherapy agents will work better for some patients and not others. People with metastatic cancer, whose tumors have what are considered normal KRAS genes, respond significantly better to two chemotherapy agents Cetuximab and Panitumumab. However, patients who have altered (or mutated) KRAS genes, do not respond to these agents.

The KRAS gene is a protein that is involved regulating cell division. Some tumors have proteins, called epidermal growth factor receptors that are found on the surface of tumors; these proteins help cancer grow. The agents Cetuximab and Panitumumab work by inhibiting the cancer cells' growth.

KRAS testing involves doing a laboratory analysis on sample tissues after surgery. About 60 percent of individuals are believed to have normal KRAS genes, while 40 percent have altered KRAS genes.

• Avoid coffee, tea, alcohol, and sugary foods.

If diarrhea persists for more than twenty-four hours, contact your doctor. Do not take any over-the-counter medication for diarrhea without consulting your doctor.

Nausea and Vomiting

Nausea and vomiting are *not* very common side effects of chemotherapy used to treat colorectal cancer. If you should experience these side effects, your oncologist can prescribe medications that will help. If vomiting persists for twenty-four hours, notify your doctor. You may need to be admitted to the hospital for intravenous fluids and medication. Here are other tips for managing nausea and vomiting:

- Take anti-nausea medications as directed.
- Breathe deeply and slowly when you feel nauseous.
- Drink six to eight glasses of water daily.
- Eat small, frequent meals rather than three large ones.
- Eat and drink slowly. Chew foods well.
- Avoid rich, spicy foods.
- Suck on ice cubes, mints, or ginger candies (unless you have mouth sores).

Some people find that the smell of food cooking bothers them. If the smell of food makes the nausea worse, try staying out of the kitchen while food is being cooked.

Hair Loss

Chemotherapy can affect hair follicles, causing temporary hair loss. Although hair loss can occur anywhere on the body, it is mainly confined to the head. During chemotherapy, some people wear hats, scarves, or wigs to cover their heads and stay warm. To cope with hair loss, try these suggestions:

- Use mild shampoos.
- Use a soft hair brush.
- Use low heat on your hair dryer.
- Don't use brush rollers to set your hair.
- Don't dye your hair or get a permanent.
- Have your hair cut short. A shorter style will make hair look thicker and fuller.
- Protect your scalp from the sun with a hat, scarf, or sunscreen.

Once treatments are complete, hair grows back. It may grow back a slightly different color or texture.

Neuropathy

Chemotherapy can cause *neuropathy*, which is damage to nerve endings. When this occurs, you may have pain, numbness, or tingling sensations in various parts of the body; the severity of these side effects depends on the amount of the chemotherapy agent you received and how quickly it was administered.

Commonly, neuropathy occurs in the hands and feet; it may interfere with activities such as buttoning a shirt, typing, writing, or playing a musical instrument. It's important to report these side effects to your oncologist right away, so he or she can adjust or suspend treatment before side effects become severe.

Neuropathy can also occur in the mouth, throat, or chest. This may result in abnormal tongue sensations, choking sensations, or sensation of pressure on your chest.

Neuropathy may be either acute or chronic. Acute neuropathy goes away within days of a chemotherapy treatment. However, chronic neuropathy can persist for weeks to months.

Cold temperatures are more likely to aggravate acute neuropathy. To help manage side effects, try these tips:

- Avoid cold drinks.
- Avoid handling cold objects.
- Inhale cold air, which may help with symptoms in the mouth and throat.

Neuropathy symptoms may be constant, or they may come and go. The chronic form may become irreversible if treatment continues, so oncologists usually reduce the dosages of the chemotherapy agent or stop the treatment. Medications are also available to alleviate neuropathy pain.

Infections

Chemotherapy can damage cells in the bone marrow, which is important to infection-fighting white blood cells. When your white blood cell count is low, it may lead to a weakening of the immune system, a condition known as *neutropenia*. This condition makes you susceptible to infections. These can include, blood infections, urinary infections, skin infections, and pneumonia. Fortunately, infection is not one of the most common side effects of chemotherapy for colorectal cancer.

However, be alert for the signs of infection—fever over 100 degrees, shaking, chills, sweats, coughing up dark or bloody sputum, pain or burning with urination, and pain or redness around cuts. Infections can be effectively treated with antibiotics. To reduce your risk of infection, take these precautions:

- Wash your hands often during the day, especially after using the bathroom.

- Avoid anyone who has a cold, flu, measles, or chicken pox.
- Stay away from children who have recently received vaccinations.
- Clean cuts and scrapes right away.
- Wear gloves when gardening or cleaning up after pets or children.
- Use a soft toothbrush that won't hurt your gums.
- Clean your rectal area gently but thoroughly after each bowel movement. Notify your doctor or nurse if this area becomes irritated or if you have hemorrhoids.

If you feel an infection coming on, notify your doctor immediately.

Fatigue

Fatigue is a common side effect of chemotherapy for colorectal cancer. Fatigue can be brought on by a low red cell count. Red blood cells deliver oxygen to the body, and if your red blood cell count is low, tissues and organs are not receiving adequate oxygen. As a result, you'll feel fatigued. This condition is called *anemia.* Most patients on chemotherapy experience some degree of fatigue. For some, fatigue occurs around the time of a treatment. Others feel fatigued during the entire course of therapy. The fatigue may last even after chemotherapy has ended, and it may take weeks for you to recover your normal energy level. For normally active patients, the fatigue can be a source of frustration or even depression. Try to stay positive and remember that the fatigue is temporary. Here are a few tips for coping with fatigue:

- Limit your activities. Do only those things that are most important to you.
- Take several short naps or breaks during the day.
- Try taking short walks or exercising lightly.

- Maintain good nutrition. Try to eat a well-balanced diet.
- Ask for help when you need it.

If your red blood cell count drops too low, you may need a blood transfusion or medication that stimulates production of red blood cells.

Impaired Blood Clotting

Chemotherapy can also cause a condition called *thrombocytopenia*, which means low blood platelet counts. Platelets are the cells that help blood to clot. Mild cases may produce no symptoms. However, if platelet counts drop low enough, symptoms may include easy bruising, which means bleeding has occurred in the small blood vessels under the skin. Shallow bleeding in the skin can also cause a purplish rash on the hands and feet. Other symptoms include spontaneous nosebleeds. In serious cases, internal bleeding may occur.

There are no medications for this condition, and physicians will usually delay or suspend chemotherapy treatment when blood platelet counts are low. This break in treatment gives the platlet count time to increase on its own. When counts drop dangerously low, blood platelet transfusions may be needed to avoid bleeding complications.

Once the course of chemotherapy has ended, the low blood counts are treatable and reversible. Throughout your treatment, your doctor will check your blood counts with blood tests.

Mouth Sores

Chemotherapy can cause painful sores and ulcers on the lips, mouth, gums, and throat. The medical term for such mouth sores is *stomatitis*. In addition to discomfort, mouth sores may make eating and drinking difficult, which may lead to dehydration. In some instances, these sores become infected. Fortunately, mouth sores disappear once the treatments have concluded. Ask your doctor about medication to treat these sores.

Stay hydrated by drinking plenty of water. Avoid spicy, sauce-based foods. Eat soft foods such as baby food, milk shakes, smoothies, yogurt, cooled oatmeal, mashed veggies, and ice cream until your condition improves. Here are additional suggestions for coping with mouth sores:

- Practice good oral hygiene—brush and floss.
- Use a soft-bristle brush to avoid irritating gum tissue.
- Avoid mouthwashes that contain a lot of salt or alcohol.
- If possible, have your teeth cleaned and any dental work completed before starting chemotherapy.
- Try sucking on ice chips; it may be soothing.

Some individuals find relief with a homemade gargle: Mix one-half teaspoon of salt and one teaspoon of baking soda in one quart of water, and gargle every four hours.

Hand-Foot Syndrome

Chemotherapy may also cause a side effect called *hand-foot syndrome*. This syndrome occurs when small amounts of chemotherapy leak out of small blood vessels and cause damage to the surrounding tissues. Symptoms typically show up in the hands and feet and include redness, swelling, blisters, and flaking skin. If symptoms become severe, they can impair walking and hand function. Your doctor will likely prescribe topical ointments for this condition. Here are other measures that may help:

- Limit use of hot water on hands and feet.
- Take cool baths.
- Pat skin dry after bathing; do not rub skin.
- Use ice packs for no more than fifteen minutes at a time. Never apply ice directly to skin—wrap the ice in a cloth.
- Apply skin-care creams as recommended by your

doctor.
- Avoid exposure to direct sunlight.
- Avoid activities, such as brisk exercise, that may cause clothing to rub against skin.

Although hand-foot syndrome typically affects hands and/ or feet, it can also occur on the elbows and knees.

Rash

Another potential side effect of some chemotherapy is an acne-like rash, called *acneiform rash*. This rash may appear around the nose, or on the face, chest, or back. Interestingly, the rash is an indication that the chemotherapy is working. Your physician may prescribe antibiotics pills or topical gels to treat the rash. Over-the-counter medications to relieve itching may also be recommended.

Changes in Skin and Nails

Changes can occur in the skin and nails during chemotherapy. Skin reactions may include drying, cracking, or peeling. Also, skin may become *hyperpigmented*, meaning the skin may darken. This may happen all over the body or in spots, causing blotches and discoloration. When a change in skin color occurs, it usually appears about two to three weeks after chemotherapy treatment begins. When treatment ends, the discoloration usually goes away as new skin cells grow. Sometimes, however, the darkening is permanent. It's important to wear sunblock when exposed to sunlight.

Nails may become discolored, and depressions may develop in both the fingernails and toenails. Once treatment is over and the nails resume normal growth, these depressions should disappear.

Allergic Reaction

An allergic reaction to a chemotherapy agent is not common, but it can occur. Symptoms of such a reaction include shortness of breath, wheezing, hoarseness, swelling, hives, and itching. These symptoms may occur within seconds of beginning a treatment, or they may occur a few hours or days later. If a reaction occurs outside your treatment center, you should contact your physician immediately. Medications can be given to counteract allergic reactions. More severe allergic reactions may lower blood pressure or cause heart attack, shock, or loss of consciousness. If you have an allergic reaction to a chemotherapy agent, it is not likely that your oncologist will use that agent again.

Infertility

Colorectal cancer mostly affects men and women who are older and no longer in their childbearing years. However, when younger cancer patients undergo chemotherapy for colorectal cancer, their fertility can be affected. This side effect is rare, but it is possible for women to have damage to their ovaries, while men may suffer damage to the delicate lining of the testicles, where sperm is produced. Among those whose fertility is affected, some women and men are eventually able to conceive; others are not. You'll want to speak with your oncologist if infertility is an issue.

Damage to the Liver and Kidneys

Chemotherapy drugs may cause damage to the liver and kidneys. The liver's primary function is to filter toxic substances from the body. If the liver is damaged, these toxins can build up and cause more liver damage. However, once chemotherapy is stopped, other drugs can be given to lessen the effects of liver damage.

The kidneys filter waste from the blood. It's not common, but chemotherapy can damage the blood vessels in the kidneys, causing them to malfunction. This malfunction is called *acute renal failure*. Fortunately, kidney damage is usually reversible.

When chemotherapy is stopped, other measures can be taken to clear toxins from the blood, allowing the kidneys time to recover.

Those who have liver or kidney disease are generally not good candidates for chemotherapy since the treatment can further damage these organs.

Memory and Thinking Impairment

Some people have temporary changes in their memory or thinking process as side effects of chemotherapy. Sometimes referred to as "chemo brain" or "brain fog," these impairments are usually mild, but can be frustrating. You might feel confused, have problems concentrating, or have trouble finding the right word you want to use to express yourself. These side effects may linger for months or possibly years. The severity of such side effects depends on how much chemotherapy was given and the length of time it was given.

If you find yourself coping with this side effect, here are steps you can take:

- Keep a note pad handy to make notes to yourself.
- Keep a calendar nearby for scheduling events.
- Get plenty of rest.
- Ask for support from family members and friends.

Some patients use exercise, music therapy, art, and reading to help overcome the mental impairments; however, it's not yet scientifically known how effective these activities are in overcoming the impairments.

Living with Chemotherapy Side Effects

As you read through the list of potential side effects, the idea of undergoing chemotherapy can be worrisome. However, most people tolerate chemotherapy with only mild to moderate side effects. Most colorectal cancer patients report that their chemotherapy was not as bad as they had thought it would be.

6 Radiation Therapy

Radiation therapy is an important tool in treating many cancers, including colorectal cancer. Patients undergoing radiation therapy today benefit from far more advanced medical technologies than were available a generation ago.

Sophisticated scanning devices produce multidimensional pictures that help doctors pinpoint the treatment area. State-of-the-art computers calculate and deliver radiation dosages so precisely that they destroy cancer cells but cause minimal damage to healthy tissues.

Radiation therapy is overseen by a *radiation oncologist,* a physician with specialty training in treating cancer with radiation. Other team members involved in treatment include: a *medical radiation physicist,* who ensures that radiation is properly tailored to each patient; a *medical dosimetrist,* who calculates the dosage; and a radiation therapist, who typically delivers the actual treatments.

How Radiation Therapy Works

Radiation kills cells that multiply rapidly. Because cancer cells multiply in a rapid, chaotic fashion, radiation treatments can stop them from reproducing. Healthy cells may also be affected by radiation, but they are not as vulnerable to it as are

External beam radiation is delivered by a linear accelerator. Treatments are usually given five days-a-week over a period of five to eight weeks.

fast-growing cancer cells. The goal of radiation therapy is to eliminate cancer cells and spare the surrounding healthy cells; however, some damage to healthy tissues is often unavoidable. Fortunately, normal cells are able to repair themselves over time.

The most common radiation treatment option for colorectal cancer is *external beam radiation therapy*, or *EBRT*. This type of treatment sends radiation rays into a tumor from outside the body. A high-energy X-ray unit called a *linear accelerator (LINAC)*, generates the beams, which target the tumor while sparing normal tissues and skin.

Radiation Therapy for Colon Cancer

Radiation therapy is often used as a follow-up treatment after surgery for colon cancer, with the intention of killing any cancer cells that may remain after the removal of a primary tumor. Radiation therapy may also be recommended if the cancer has attached to a neighboring organ, such as the kidney, bladder, or spleen, or has infiltrated the lining of the abdomen. Postoperative radiation therapy may also be combined with chemotherapy.

Radiation Therapy for Rectal Cancer

Radiation therapy plays a routine role in treating rectal cancer. Radiation is frequently used prior to surgery to shrink the tumor so it can be removed through the anus rather than through a more extensive abdominal incision. Shrinking the tumor first with radiation increases the chances of destroying the cancer completely. In fact, research shows that the risk of recurrence over the next ten years is cut by 50 percent when patients receive radiation therapy to the rectal area prior to surgery.

In addition, your doctor may recommend radiation therapy after surgery to kill any cancer cells that may remain.

Before Your First Treatment

Before your first radiation treatment, you will have a simulation appointment with your radiation therapy team. This is a planning session during which they will determine where the radiation beams will be directed and how your body will be positioned for each treatment.

During the simulation, you'll be asked to lie on a treatment table, most likely on your back. You'll be fitted with an immobilization device; it is a comfortable, yet rigid, cradle that holds your body in place during each treatment session. The immobilization device is created by pouring resin or polystyrene beads into a bag made of urethane, nylon or another sturdy material. The bag is then molded to the specific contours of your body.

You may be injected with a contrast fluid, which will show up in tissues when you undergo a body scan. This scan, which gives your doctor a detailed view of the tumor and the surrounding healthy tissues, pinpoints the part of the body to be treated.

After the treatment area is defined and filmed, technologist will mark your outer skin area with tiny tattoos. These tiny marks serve as a "map" that tells the radiation therapist where to direct the radiation beam during treatments. (The tattoos appear as tiny freckles and most patients do not find them bothersome.)

Receiving a Radiation Treatment

During a treatment, you lie on a treatment table while the arm of the linear accelerator circles your body, sending calculated radiation doses to the tumor.

External beam radiation therapy is typically administered five days a week over five to eight weeks. Each treatment lasts a few minutes, but the preparation can take up to thirty minutes. The treatments are spread over time because the total dosage necessary to kill a tumor would cause too much damage to normal tissues if given at once. You need time for your healthy cells to repair themselves.

Types of Radiation Therapy

Three-Dimensional
Conformal Radiation Therapy (3D-CRT)

A type of external beam radiation therapy, *three-dimensional conformal radiation therapy (3D-CRT)* is an advanced technology used in many medical facilities to treat colorectal cancer. It involves the use of special CT scanners and computers to map the tumor in three-dimensional form and then match, or conform, beams to the cancer's unique shape. Once the outline is calculated, the radiation is aimed at the tumor from multiple angles.

A specialized form of 3D-CRT known as *intensity modulated radiation therapy (IMRT)* also shows promise for treatment of colorectal cancer. Besides conforming radiation beams to an individual mass, IMRT allows radiation oncologists to break up each beam into smaller "beamlets" and adjust them in intensity, or strength. With such capability, doctors can deliver an even higher dose of radiation to the tumor while minimizing damage to nearby healthy tissues. Although IMRT is offered at many medical centers, some insurers won't cover the cost.

Image-Guided Radiation Therapy (IGRT)

Another form of radiation treatment, *image-guided radiation therapy (IGRT)*, uses images, such as X-rays or CT scans, to help radiation oncologists deliver the radiation beam more precisely. Since tumors and healthy tissues can move between treatments, viewing these areas allows physicians to make corrections and tailor the beam's focus. During IGRT, the doctor "fuses" the images taken prior to the start of therapy with new images taken that day, to see if adjustments must be made. Available at many medical centers, IGRT is used to treat both colon and rectal cancers.

Intraoperative Radiation Therapy (IORT)

Another form of radiation treatment, *intraoperative radiation therapy (IORT)* is used to deliver a dose of intense radiation to a tumor during surgery. After the surgeon removes as much of the mass as possible, a linear accelerator delivers a concentrated, high-dose beam directly to the remaining part of the tumor or the area from which the tumor has been removed. Although IORT shows promise for colon and anal cancers, the technology is not commonly used. It's currently available at only a few medical centers. In these locations, it's used to treat malignancies that either are attached to vital tissues or can't be removed entirely. The treatment is also effective for tumors that can't be cured with surgery alone or that will likely recur in the same area.

Brachytherapy/Endocavitary Radiation Therapy

Also called *internal radiation therapy, brachytherapy* involves the use of radioactive pellets that are inserted next to or directly into a tumor. Although brachytherapy has a limited role in treating colon cancer, it's used somewhat routinely in treating rectal cancer.

Endocavitary radiation therapy, a specialized form of brachytherapy, is effective in the treatment of small, early-stage rectal cancers. In this procedure, a high dose of radiation is administered through the rectum. The advantage of this endocavitary approach is that the radiation reaches the rectum without passing through the skin or tissues of the abdomen.

The patient is usually awake during these radiation treatments, which take about twenty minutes each. The treatment is repeated several times over a two-week period. The procedure is usually performed at larger hospitals but may also be offered at some community hospitals.

Side Effects of Radiation Therapy

Radiation treatments are not painful—most patients don't feel anything during a radiation treatment. Yet the beams can affect any skin, muscle, and intra-abdominal organs in its path. This can produce symptoms ranging from skin irritation to changes in bowel movements. Although side effects can be distressing, most symptoms are treatable. They usually disappear after therapy, although some symptoms may be permanent. Also, keep in mind that not everyone experiences every side effect.

Skin Irritation

Skin irritation is the most common side effect of radiation therapy. As treatment progresses, any skin in the beam's path may become dry, irritated, and peel like a sunburn. The changes may leave the skin permanently rough and darkened. You can minimize any irritation during treatment, however, by taking these measures:

- Wear loose, soft clothing over the treated area.
- Avoid any lotion, soap, or powder on the area within

four hours just before treatment.
- Ask your doctor or nurse about lotions or creams that may help after treatment.
- Avoid rubbing, scratching, or scrubbing the treated skin.
- Bathe in lukewarm water.

Loss of Appetite

Because the beams can be hard on the lining of your gastrointestinal tract, radiation can affect your appetite, particularly if you're being treated for colon cancer. Rectal cancer patients usually don't experience a loss of appetite. In either case, however, it's important to maintain a nutritious diet so your body will stay energized. If you lose your appetite, here are some suggestions to follow:
- Eat smaller, more frequent meals, including healthful snacks.
- Avoid fatty foods.
- Work with a dietitian to develop a plan that helps you maintain or gain weight.

Diarrhea and Nausea

Diarrhea is a common side effect of radiation therapy for both colon and rectal cancer. Because the bowel and stomach are sensitive to radiation, they may become inflamed, triggering abdominal symptoms. You may experience bloating, cramps, and chronic diarrhea, or frequent bowel movements. If you're undergoing treatment for colon cancer, you may also have bouts of nausea. Fortunately, by being proactive, you can alleviate such symptoms. In the case of diarrhea, follow these measures:
- Increase your intake of fluids, such as broth. Drink at least six eight-ounce glasses of fluids daily, since persistent diarrhea can cause your body to lose water and nutrients.

- Avoid caffeine (such as coffee and tea) and alcohol-containing drinks, since they lead to fluid loss.
- Avoid foods that intensify diarrhea: milk products, nuts, seeds, raw high-fiber vegetables (such as corn, cauliflower, and broccoli), and fruits with skins.
- Choose foods low in fiber, such as bananas, applesauce, rice, and toast.
- Tell your doctor if you have watery, loose stools more than two or three times a day or notice mucus or blood in the stool.

If you have diarrhea, your doctor may prescribe an anti-diarrhea medication. Don't take over-the-counter medications without consulting your physician.

You can minimize nausea by avoiding sweet, fried, spicy, or fatty foods and substituting bland items, such as dry crackers and flat ginger ale. It helps to eat smaller, more frequent meals. Also, eat foods at room temperature if the odor of hot foods upsets your stomach. Other tips include:

- Breathe deeply and slowly when you feel nauseous.
- Learn relaxation exercises to help you feel less anxious and more in control.
- Ask your doctor about medications or other devices, such as wrist acupressure bands, that may decrease the problem.

Bowel function usually returns to normal after treatment is completed. However, some people notice more frequent bowel movements and/or loose stools after radiation treatment; these changes can last indefinitely.

Bladder Irritation

Because the bladder is close to the rectum, radiation therapy may affect this organ, potentially causing infection, burning when urinating, or even blood in the urine. You may feel like you have to urinate when you really don't need to. Bladder irritation is rarely a permanent side effect.

Rectal Irritation

When radiation is directed at a rectal tumor, inflammation is a common side effect. You may experience itching or burning pain during bowel movements. Your rectum also may be sore if your bowels are moving frequently. In either case, there are steps you can take to relieve the discomfort:

- Take sitz baths—sit in a few inches of warm water.
- Pat your rectal area dry with a soft cloth after cleansing.
- Ask your doctor about safe and effective creams and suppositories.

The affected area should heal after treatment has ended. Permanent rectal discomfort can occur, but it's infrequent.

Fatigue

Many patients report being tired during radiation therapy, particularly as the treatments progress. Treatment takes time, during which your energy levels will be lower than normal. You may feel slightly tired, or you may suffer from extreme weariness. However, the fatigue should diminish within weeks of finishing treatment. Until then, you can counter your low energy by following these suggestions:

- Take short rests when you feel tired. Avoid long naps so you sleep well at night, and move slowly when you lie down or sit up to avoid dizziness.
- Do mild exercise; add a brisk twenty-minute walk to your daily routine.
- Take in sufficient calories; poor eating habits can add to fatigue, but a healthful diet can help immeasurably.
- Drink plenty of liquids; drinking six to eight glasses of water daily helps you stay hydrated and energized as well.

During treatment, it's also a good idea to focus on important tasks; don't spend energy on tasks that can wait. If your fatigue is severe or chronic, ask for help with routine daily chores, or prioritize what needs to be done.

Infections

Radiation can cause a reduction in your white blood cell count. (White blood cells fight infection.) This effect is much more likely, however, when radiation and chemotherapy are delivered at the same time. Without sufficient white blood cells, your body can't fight infections adequately. Because it's important to stay healthy during your therapy, be sure to take these measures:

- Wash your hands often to kill germs.
- Avoid people with colds, and avoid crowds. Also avoid children who've been recently vaccinated with live viruses.
- Protect yourself against cuts and open sores that could become infected.
- Call your doctor immediately if you develop any signs of an infection: severe chills, a cough, a temperature of 100.5°F or higher, or pain during urination.

Whatever your side effects might be from radiation therapy, it's important to remember that they can be managed, if not eliminated completely. With guidance from your medical team, you can address most of the problems successfully.

Living with Radiation Therapy Side Effects

As with chemotherapy, side effects of radiation therapy for colorectal cancer can be managed. Still, it is important to be aware of the side effects that you may experience so you can report them to your oncologist right away. The sooner your physician knows about side effects, the sooner he or she can take steps to alleviate them.

7 Follow-up Care

After you've been treated for colorectal cancer, your physician will monitor you closely for any signs of cancer recurrence. You will be scheduled for periodic examinations for the next few years.

Follow-up treatment typically involves examinations every three to six months for the first two to three years, and then every six months for the next two years. If you have been treated for an early-stage cancer, you may not require monitoring as frequently. Follow-up examinations will include several diagnostic tests.

Diagnostic Tests

The tests you'll undergo as part of your follow-up care are the same types of diagnostic tests you had prior to your treatment. They involve blood tests, X-rays, scans, and colonoscopies.

Blood Tests

Routine blood tests will also measure your levels of two proteins, *carcinoembryonic antigen (CEA)* and *carbohydrate antigen (CA) 19-9*. Often referred to as *tumor markers*, both proteins shed colorectal cancer cells into the bloodstream. Doctors test the levels of these markers prior to treatment, and usually find that elevated levels go down after treatment. However, if levels go back up again, it may be a sign that the cancer has recurred. If your doctor finds high levels of these proteins, he or she will perform other tests to investigate further. Your doctor may order these blood tests every three months for the first three years.

Note that elevated levels of these tumor markers in the blood does *not* always mean cancer has recurred. Increased levels may also be symptoms of noncancerous conditions, such as gallstones, rectal polyps, inflammation, cirrhosis, peptic ulcers, pancreatitis, ulcerative colitis, emphysema, and benign breast disease.

Imaging Tests

Imaging tests allow your physician to view your internal organs. Such tests may include CT scans, PET scans, MRI scans, bone scans, or ultrasound scans. If your doctor determines that you have a higher risk for colon cancer recurrence, he or she may schedule routine scans of your chest and abdomen. If there is a risk for recurrence of rectal cancer, your physician will likely schedule scans of your pelvis. These tests are typically recommended once a year for the first three years.

Colonoscopy

Your physician will want you to have regular colonoscopies that will check for polyps or any new tumors. A colonoscopy is usually recommended in the first year after surgery, then once every three years. If these tests show no signs of cancer, the next colonoscopy is usually recommended at five years. The frequency of the colonoscopies is related to the nature of your risk for recurrence.

Cancer Recurrence

What if the cancer recurs? This is the question that lingers in the minds of most cancer patients and their families. Your risk of recurrence is directly related to the stage of your cancer at the time of the initial diagnosis. A cancer caught early and confined to the colorectal wall is less likely to recur than a cancer that has spread to surrounding tissue or lymph nodes at the time of initial diagnosis. If colorectal cancer recurs, it usually does so within the first five years after diagnosis and treatment. Recurrent cancer is divided into three categories. When cancer recurs very near the same site as the original cancer, it is called a *local recurrence*. It is a *regional recurrence* if the cancer is found in lymph nodes and tissues near the original site. If the cancer recurs in other parts of the body, it is considered a *distant recurrence*. The liver is the most common organ in which colorectal cancer recurs.

Once you've finished your initial treatments and it's time to see your physician for a follow-up examination, you may be anxious, especially in the beginning; however, most people report that they become less anxious as time goes on.

Symptoms of Cancer Recurrence

It is important to stay alert for any symptoms of cancer recurrence so that it can be diagnosed and treated early. The symptoms of a recurring colorectal cancer are similar to the symptoms of an initial colorectal cancer.

- *Change in bowel habits:* Prolonged constipation not responsive to laxatives, abdominal pain, persistent diarrhea, or a change in stool characteristics.
- *Rectal bleeding:* Passing dark or bright red blood with bowel movements, or a change in stool color.
- *Persistent urge to have a bowel movement:* Urge to have a bowel movement despite just having had a bowel movement.
- *Excess mucus secretion:* With bowel movements.
- *Chronic abdominal pain, bloating, and fullness:* Persistant discomfort that does not go away with medications.

- *Decreased appetite, weight loss, and fatigue:* Possible signs of a recurrence in the liver or other organs.
- *Jaundice:* A yellowing of the eyes or skin, which may indicate a recurrence in the liver.
- *New joint or bone pain:* Onset of acute back or rib pain may be a symptom of a recurrence in the spine.

Treatment for Recurring Cancer

If your colorectal cancer does return, there are treatment options, depending on the nature of the recurrence. Options include surgery, chemotherapy, radiation therapy, or a combination of these treatments. Other potential treatments include cryoablation, radiofrequency ablation, and portal vein infusion.

Surgery

If your surgeon determines you are a candidate for surgery, another operation may be the best measure. Surgery has the best chance of being successful if the recurrent tumor is isolated to one organ and confined to one area. If, for instance, you have a solitary tumor that is confined to one part of your liver, surgery to remove a portion of your liver may be the best option. Or, if you have a single tumor that is confined to a single area of your lung, surgery may be an option. If the cancer has returned in a different part of your colon, then, again, surgery may be the best option.

Cryoablation and Radiofrequency Ablation

If colorectal cancer returns in several areas of one organ, such as the liver, then surgery is not the best treatment. In this case, cryoablation and radiofrequency ablation are possible options. *Cryoablation* is a minimally invasive surgical procedure that can be performed on an outpatient basis. It involves the placement of a probe into the middle of the tumor and first freezing it with liquid nitrogen. Once the tumor is frozen, heat is immediately applied to thaw it. The combination of freezing and thawing is effective for killing tumor cells without harming normal surrounding cells. The procedure usually is completed in two to three hours.

Radiofrequency ablation kills cancer cells with intense heat generated by high-frequency radio waves. During the procedure, a physician inserts a needle electrode directly into a tumor. The electrode emits heat that destroys cancer cells. This treatment is also a minimally invasive procedure that is often performed on an outpatient basis; the procedure may take ten to thirty minutes. More than one treatment may be required for large tumors.

Chemotherapy

If your cancer recurrence involves multiple organs, chemotherapy in combination with radiation therapy may be the best option. If you have undergone chemotherapy previously, your oncologist will likely prescribe different chemotherapy drugs for the next round of treatments.

In the case of a liver metastasis, chemotherapy can be directly infused in the liver; this direct infusion, called a *hepatic artery infusion,* is given through a catheter that is surgically inserted into the main artery that enters the liver. This approach has proven more effective in prolonging survival and reducing recurrence compared to standard chemotherapy treatments.

When you have begun chemotherapy treatments after a recurrence, your medical oncologist will monitor your progress during chemotherapy. Diagnostic scans, such as CT scans and PET scans, and blood tests will be performed to assess your response to the chemotherapy. If your condition has improved, your oncologist will likely continue the same treatment. If tests show the chemotherapy isn't working effectively against the cancer, your oncologist may switch you to another chemotherapy drug.

Radiation Therapy

Radiation therapy may be used alone for a recurrence of either colon or rectal cancer, depending on the goal of the treatment. The goal may be to limit local control of the cancer, to treat an obstruction, or to control bleeding or pain.

If the patient can tolerate chemotherapy, it may be combined with radiation therapy to strengthen the treatment. In some cases, intraoperative radiation therapy may be an option. As mentioned earlier, in this procedure, a radiation beam is aimed directly at a tumor during surgery. This approach can be more effective than standard external beam radiation. A combination of radiation and chemotherapy may be recommended if surgery is not possible.

Clinical Trials

Your oncologist may recommend participation in a clinical trial. These trials may be part of a person's initial treatment. Or, they may be recommended after standard treatments have failed. A clinical trial is a research study, conducted with patients, that applies new treatments or new combinations of treatments to those chosen to participate. Many of today's best standard treatments were first available to patients in clinical trials.

It is important to remember that participants in clinical trials do *not* receive untested treatments. Participants are not treated as "human guinea pigs." New treatments are offered to patients in clinical trials only after extensive laboratory research has demonstrated that these treatments are at least as good as, and potentially much better than, standard therapies.

Participating in a Clinical Trial

Participation in a clinical trial is strictly voluntary. You may stop participating in a clinical trial at any time before, during, or after you have received the new treatment. Upon leaving the trial, if any medical problems result from the trial treatment, you will continue to receive appropriate medical care.

How do you enroll in a trial? Researchers set guidelines for who is eligible to participate in a clinical trial. These guidelines include factors such as age, sex, type and stage of disease, previous treatment history, and other medical conditions. Ask your doctor or oncologist to help you find a trial that is suitable. He or she will ask you to sign a consent form after reviewing all the details of the clinical trial with you, including the potential benefits and risks.

Benefits and Risks of Clinical Trials

There are potential benefits and risks to participating in a clinical trial. The National Cancer Institute lists the benefits and risks as follows:

Potential Benefits
- Health care is provided by leading physicians in the field of cancer research.
- You receive access to new drugs and interventions before they are widely available.
- Your health is closely monitored.
- You have a more active role in your own health care.
- If the approach being studied is found to be helpful, you may be among the first to benefit.
- The trial is an opportunity to make a valuable contribution to cancer research.

Potential Risks
- Despite research on new drugs and procedures, it's possible that the treatments may have side effects or risks unknown to the doctors.
- New drugs and procedures may be ineffective or may be less effective than current approaches.
- Even if a new approach has benefits, it may not work for you.

Where to Find Clinical Trials

Clinical trials are offered in hospitals, cancer centers,

doctors' offices, and clinics throughout the United States and internationally. However, some trials are available only at certain locations. Clinical trials are sponsored by a number of organizations, both public and private. The National Cancer Institute sponsors many clinical trials and works with other organizations that sponsor clinical trials. You'll find Web site information about the National Cancer Institute in the Resources section at the back of this book.

8   Prevention and Early Detection

Studies have repeatedly shown that annual screening for colorectal cancer prolongs survival and saves lives. In fact, annual screening actually reduces your risk of getting colorectal cancer by up to 20 percent—when precancerous polyps are found, they can be removed before they become cancerous. Unfortunately, today only about 40 percent of Americans undergo any type of routine screening. As a result, colorectal cancer remains the third leading cause of cancer death in the United States.

Screening according to Risk Factors

How often should you be screened for colorectal cancer? The frequency of screening depends on whether you have an average, increased, or high risk for developing the disease. Those in the average risk category are those with no known risk factors; this includes nearly 75 percent of Americans.

Average Risk

If you are at average risk, you should start undergoing routine screening once you reach the age of fifty. The following screening tests are recommended:

- A fecal occult blood test every year. This test checks for hidden blood in stool samples.
- A flexible sigmoidoscopy every five years. This test examines the interior walls of the rectum and the

lower third of the colon. The majority of cancers start in this area.

- A colonoscopy every ten years. This test examines the entire length of the colon.

Increased Risk

Individuals are considered at increased risk if they have a history of polyps (*adenomas*) that can become cancerous; have had colon or rectal cancer; have a first-degree relative (parent, brother, sister, or child) who has had colorectal cancer or adenomas; or have two or more second-degree relatives (aunt, uncle, grandparent) who have had colorectal cancer. These are the recommendations for screening:

- Colonoscopy is the only screening test that should be recommended.
- In the case of a family history of cancer or adenomas in a first=degree relative, your first colonoscopy should be done at age forty or ten years earlier than the age of the youngest relative when he or she was diagnosed with colorectal cancer. For example, if your father was diagnosed with colorectal cancer at age forty-five, you should begin having routine colonoscopies at age thirty-five.

Colonoscopy recommendations for individuals at increased risk of colorectal cancer vary based on factors such as how many polyps they have and the size of the polyps. If you're in this group, talk with your doctor about when to begin colonoscopy screening and how often it should be repeated.

High Risk

You are considered at high risk for colorectal cancer if you have a personal history of inflammatory bowel disease, including Crohn's disease and ulcerative colitis, of sufficient duration—at least eight years. You are also at high risk if you have a family history of hereditary colorectal cancer. The two types of this cancer are familial adenomatous polyposis (FAP) and hereditary nonpolyposis colon cancer (HNPCC), discussed in chapter 1.

If you are at high risk, talk to your doctor about how often you should be screened. The frequency of screening depends on the type of risk factor you have. Here are the guidelines:

- If you have inflammatory bowel disease, Crohn's disease, or ulcerative colitis, routine colonoscopies are recommended every one to two years. Talk with your doctor about how soon after the onset of the disease you should start the colonoscopies. Also ask about undergoing a tissue biopsy to check for any abnormal cells in the lining of the colon.
- If you have familial adenomatous polypsis, get a flexible sigmoidoscopy or colonoscopy every six to twelve months once you reach puberty.
- If you have hereditary nonpolyposis colon cancer syndrome, experts recommend a colonoscopy every two years starting at age twenty-five. This should continue until you reach age forty. Thereafter, schedule a colonoscopy every year.

Genetic Testing

An estimated 5 to 10 percent of all colorectal cancers involve inherited genes. If you have a strong family history of colorectal cancer, such as several members diagnosed before age sixty, genetic tests are now available that can predict your risk of developing the disease later in life.

These genetic tests involve sampling your blood to test for gene mutations, which are abnormal genes. If you test positive for these genetic mutations, you have an 80 percent higher risk than the average person of developing colorectal cancer as you get older. If you have familial adenomatous polyposis or hereditary nonpolyposis colon cancer, you have a 50 percent chance of passing the abnormal gene on to each of your children.

By knowing your risk, you and your doctor can develop an aggressive screening program that can detect cancer early or prevent it altogether.

Lifestyle Factors and Colorectal Cancer

Several lifestyle factors can influence the development of colorectal cancer. These factors include diet, body weight, exercise, smoking, and the use of supplements and medications.

Proper Nutrition

Diet plays a major role in our health. Some studies show that diet is a factor in the development of colorectal cancer. It is well known that colorectal cancer is primarily a disease of Western industrialized countries such as the United States and Canada. The lifetime risk of getting the disease in Western countries is 6 percent, but the incidence is much lower in countries such as Japan, where much less red meat and fat are consumed. According to some studies, by adhering to a healthful diet, you can reduce your risk of colorectal cancer by up to 50 percent.

Reducing your intake of processed and red meat, cholesterol, and saturated fatty acids can help prevent precancerous polyps and colorectal cancer. A diet high in fruits and vegetables may also help prevent the formation of polyps and cancer. Fruits and green, leafy vegetables contain antioxidants that protect cells against cancer-causing agents in our diet and in the environment. Antioxidants include vitamins A, C, and E. Carotenoids, lycopene, and lutein are other antioxidants commonly found in fruits and vegetables.

It's also believed that fiber helps prevent colorectal cancer. Fiber promotes good bowel function, dilutes carcinogens in our diet that ultimately make their way to the colon, and decreases the time the inner lining of the colon is exposed to carcinogens.

Some studies have suggested that a diet deficient in calcium increases your risk of developing polyps and colorectal cancer. One study showed a 20 percent reduction in the incidence of colorectal cancer in patients taking calcium supplements. Calcium appears to block the effects of some carcinogens found in the colon and helps prevent polyp and cancer formation. Vitamin D may also help guard against colorectal cancer since it helps the body absorb calcium.

Alcohol consumption may also be a factor in the development of colorectal cancer. It's believed that consuming more than three alcoholic drinks a day increases the risk of forming large polyps.

Body Weight and Exercise

Obesity is linked to colorectal cancer in both men and women, but the link seems to be stronger in men. Some studies show that carrying extra fat around the waist increases the risk of colorectal cancer.

Studies also confirm the benefits of daily vigorous exercise in preventing colorectal cancer. Daily exercise is helpful in preventing many other diseases as well, such as heart and lung disease. Try to get at least thirty minutes of exercise, such as brisk walking, every day.

Smoking

It's a fact that smoking causes lung cancer, and it may also contribute to other cancers, including colorectal cancer. As technology to analyze the DNA in genes becomes more advanced, the link between smoking and colorectal cancer becomes stronger. Medical data suggests that smoking can have a damaging effect on the DNA of colon cells, predisposing them to becoming cancerous. By smoking, you increase your risk for a number of noncancerous diseases as well. If you smoke, talk with your doctor about strategies to quit, including the use of prescription drugs and nicotine patches.

Hormone Therapy

There is emerging evidence that postmenopausal women who take the hormone supplements estrogen and progesterone have a reduced risk of getting colorectal cancer; however, estrogen alone does not appear to reduce the risk. This evidence comes mainly from the millions of postmenopausal women who take hormone supplements to reduce the risk of osteoporosis—weakening of the bones. However, research also links hormone therapy to heart disease, blood clots, and breast, lung, and uterine cancers.

The hormones estrogen and progesterone do not appear to lower the risk for rectal cancer.

Aspirin and Other Medications

Aspirin and similar medications can prevent the formation of polyps and colorectal cancer. Over the last three decades, several large studies have focused on people taking an aspirin a day to reduce the risk of heart disease. Surprisingly, these studies show that individuals who have taken aspirin daily for at least five years also have a 40 to 50 percent reduction in the risk of polyps and colorectal cancer. Researchers believe that aspirin somehow reverses the precancerous changes in growing precancerous polyps.

Other aspirin-like medications, including ibuprofen, have the same effect. Ibuprofen is a nonsteroidal anti-inflammatory drug (NSAID) and is primarily used to treat pain and inflammation. However, these medications also carry side effects such as possible bleeding. Ask your doctor whether you should be taking any of them.

Importance of Early Detection

As mentioned earlier, the key to prevention and early detection of colorectal cancer is routine screening. The earlier colorectal cancer is diagnosed, the better the chance for a cure.

Symptoms of an early colorectal cancer may be subtle or not noticeable at all. However, in cases that are diagnosed early, the cure rate is approximately 90 percent. Talk to your doctor about routine screenings.

Appendix

TNM Classifcation System

Doctors use an internationally recognized system for classifying the extent to which a cancer has spread. Known as the "TNM" classification system, it has been accepted by the International Union Against Cancer (UICC) and the American Joint Committee on Cancer (AJCC).

In the initials, TNM, the "T" stands for tumor—it's size and the extent of any spreading. The "N" is for lymph nodes and refers to any spread of the cancer to lymph nodes. The "M" is for metastasis or spread to other organs. Descriptions of the system are listed below.

Tumor (T)	
Tx	Primary tumor cannot be assessed
T0	No evidence of primary tumor
Tis	Carcinoma in situ: Intraepithelial or invasion of lamina propria
T1	Tumor invades submucosa
T2	Tumor invades muscularis propria
T3	Tumor invades through the muscularis propria into pericolrectal tissues
T4a	Tumor penetrates to the surface of the viscreal peritoneum
T4b	Tumor directly invades or is adherent to other organs and structures

Nodes (N)	
NX	Regional lymph nodes cannot be assessed
N0	No regional lymph node metastasis
N1	Metastasis in one to three reginal lymph nodes
N1a	Metastasis in one regional lymph node
N1b	Metastasis in two to three regional lymph nodes
N1c	Tumor deposit(s) in the subsurosa, mesentery, or nonperitonealized pericolic or perirectal tissues without regional nodal metastasis
N2	Metastasis in four or more regional lymph nodes
N2a	Metastasis in four to six regional lymph nodes
N2b	Metastasis in seven or more regional lymph nodes

Metastasis	
M0	No distant metastasis
M1	Distant metastasis
M1a	Metastasis confined to one organ or site (e.g., liver, lung, ovary, nonregional node)
M1b	Metastasis in more than one organ/site or the peritoneum

Cancer Stages with TNM Classifications

Stage	T	N	M
0	Tis	N0	M0
I	T1	N0	M0
	T2	N0	M0
IIA	T3	N0	M0
IIB	T4a	N0	M0
IIC	T4b	N0	M0
IIIA	T1-2	N1/N1c	M0
	T1	N2a	M0
IIIB	T3-T4a	N1/N1c	M0
	T2-T3	N2a	M0
	T1-T2	N2b	M0
IIIC	T4a	N2a	M0
	T3-T4a	N2b	M0
	T4b	N1-N2	M0
IVA	Any T	Any N	M1a
IVB	Any T	Any N	M2b

Resources

American Cancer Society
15999 Clifton Road NE
Atlanta, GA 30329-4251
(800) 227-2345
www.cancer.org

American College of Gastroenterology
P.O. Box 34260
Bethesda, MD 20827
(301) 263-9000
www.acg.gi.org

American College of Surgeons
633 North Saint Clair Street
Chicago, IL 60611
(312) 302-5000
www.facs.org

American Gastroenterological Association
4930 Del Ray Avenue
Bethesda, MD 20814
(301) 654-2055
www.gastro.org

American Society of Colon & Rectal Surgeons
85 West Algonquin Road, Suite 550
Arlington Heights, IL 60005
(847) 290-9184
www.fascrs.org

Cancer Care
275 7th Avenue
New York, NY 10001
(800) 813-HOPE
www.cancercare.org

Caring 4 Cancer
P4 Healthcare
3012 Oak Lawn Avenue
Dallas, TX 75219
www.caring4cancer.com

Colon Cancer Alliance
1025 Vermont Avenue NW, Suite 1066
Washington, DC 20005
(877) 442-2030
www.ccalliance.org

Colon Cancer Challenge Foundation
P.O. Box 113
Rye, NY 10580
(914) 967-8900
www.coloncancerchallenge.org

National Cancer Institute
Public Inquiries Office
6116 Executive Boulevard, Suite 300
Bethesda, MD 20892
(800) 422-6237
www.nci.nih.gov

National Coalition for Cancer Survivorship

1010 Wayne Avenue, Suite 770
Silver Spring, MD 20910
(888) 650-9127
www.canceradvocacy.org

National Comprehensive Cancer Network

275 Commerce Drive, Suite 300
Fort Washington, PA 19034
(215) 690-0300
www.nccn.com

United Ostomy Association of America, Inc.

P.O. Box 512
Northfield, MN 55057
(800) 826-0826
www.uoa.org

Wound Ostomy and Continence Nurses Society (WOCN)

15000 Commerce Parkway, Suite C
Mt. Laurel, NJ 08054
(888) 224-9626
www.wocn.org

Staying Connected to Family and Friends

The following are Web sites where you can post private health updates about yourself or a loved one.

CareFlash
www.careflash.com

MyLifeLine.org
www.mylifeline.org

CarePages
www.carepages,com

Family Patient
www.familypatient.com

CaringBridge
www.caringbridge.com

The Status
www.thestatus.com

Lotsa Helping Hands
www.lotsahelpinghands.com

Glossary

A

Acneiform rash: An acne-like reaction to some chemotherapy agents. Unlike true acne, the breakouts are sterile and contain no bacteria.

Adenocarcinoma: The most common type of colorectal cancer.

Adenoma: a benign glandular tumor which over time may become malignant.

Adjuvant therapy: Additional therapy given to supplement an initial therapy.

Ambulatory infusion pump: A small, wearable pump that delivers measured amounts of a drugs over time.

Anemia: A medical term given to the condition of a low red blood cell count.

Anesthesiologist: A doctor trained in administering anesthesia during surgery.

Anterior-posterior (AP) resection: The major curative operation for cancers of the distal rectum.

Anus: The opening at the end of the rectum where stool exits the body.

Ascending colon: The first part of the colon on the right side of the abdominal cavity.

B

Bacteremia: An infection of the blood stream caused by bacteria.

Barium enema: An X-ray test that outlines the colon wall and is used to identify polyps.

Benign: Noncancerous.

Bilirubin: A compound made by the liver and involved in digestion of food.

Biopsy: A procedure to surgically remove a piece of tissue for analysis.

Bladder: The organ, located behind the pubic bone, that collects urine.

Bone scan: A specialized X-ray test used to evaluate the skeleton for the spread of cancer.

Brachytherapy: A form of radiation therapy used to treat cancer.

C

Carcinoembryonic antigen (CEA): A protein in the blood specifically produced by cancer cells in the colon, rectum, pancreas, and breast.

Carcinoma in situ: Cells that show the earliest signs of cancerous changes.

Cecum: The beginning part of the right or ascending colon.

Chemotherapy: Therapy that uses chemical agents to treat cancer.

Colectomy: Surgery to remove all or some portion of the colon.

Colon: The organ in the body responsible for the excretion of waste.

Colonoscope: A fiber-optic, flexible scope used to perform a colonoscopy.

Colonoscopy: The procedure doctors perform to examine the inside of the colon.

Colorectal surgeon: A surgeon specifically trained to treat diseases of the colon and rectum.

Colostomy: The sewing of an open end of colon to the skin on the abdomen so stool can flow into an attached, plastic pouch.

Colostomy takedown: The reversal of colostomy, in which the large intestine is reconnected with the rectum to restore normal movement of stool.

Complete blood count (CBC): A blood test used to measure the red and white blood cells in the body.

Computerized axial tomography (CAT or CT) Scan: A specialized X-ray used to examine the internal organs.

Contrast: A liquid taken by mouth or injected into a vein to enhance the quality of X-ray pictures.

Cowden's disease: An inherited disease resulting in the formation of colorectal polyps.

Crohn's disease: An inflammatory disease of the colon wall resulting in diarrhea and pain.

Cryoablation: A process that uses extreme cold to remove tissue.

CT colonography: Often referred to as a virtual colonoscopy, a CT scan designed to simulate a colonoscopy to look for polyps and cancers.

Cystogram: An X-ray test used to evaluate the inside lining of the bladder.

D

Descending colon: The part of the colon located on the left side of the abdominal cavity and connecting to the sigmoid colon.

Diarrhea: The passing of liquid stool.

Diverticulosis: A disease of the colon characterized by the formation of small, weak pouches in the wall and resulting in constipation and pain.

Duodenum: The name given to the first part of the small intestine leading from the stomach.

Dysplastic: Precancerous changes seen in colorectal polyps.

E

Electrolytes: Blood components of sodium, potassium, chloride, and carbon dioxide.

Endocavitary radiation: A type of radiation treatment used to treat cancer.

Enterostomal nurse: A nurse specializing in the education and care of a colostomy.

Epidural catheter: A small tube inserted at the base of the back for pain control after an operation.

Esophagus: A tubelike organ that carries food from the mouth to the stomach.

External beam: A type of radiation treatment used to treat cancer.

Extramural: Referring to outside the wall of an organ.

F

Familial adenomatous polyposis (FAP): An inherited disease resulting in the formation of hundreds or thousands of precancerous polyps at an early age.

Fatigue: Tiredness.

Fecal occult blood test (FOBT): Checks for hidden blood in the stool.

Fistula: An abnormal connection between two or more hollow organs.

Fluorouracil (5-FU): A chemotherapy drug used to treat colorectal cancer.

Forceps: A surgical instrument used to grab objects.

G

Gardner's syndrome: An inherited disease resulting in the formation of precancerous colorectal polyps.

Gastroenterologist: A doctor specializing in treating diseases of the esophagus, stomach, intestine, colon, rectum, and anus.

Gastrointestinal tract: An all-encompassing term given to the organs involved in eating, digestion, absorption, and waste excretion.

General anesthesia: Anesthesia given with the purpose of putting patients to sleep during surgery.

General surgeon: A surgeon qualified to operate on a variety of diseases, including colorectal cancer.

H

Hamartoma polyp: A benign tumor that grows at the same rate as the surrounding tissue, but grows in a disorganized mass.

Hand-foot syndrome: Side effect caused be chemotherapy agents leaking through veins and injuring tissues, often in the hands and feet.

Hematocrit: Red blood cell count given as a percentage.

Hemoglobin: The level of iron present as it relates to red blood cell count.

Hemorrhoids: Abnormal veins located around the anus, causing bleeding and pain.

Hepatic artery infusion: Delivers chemotherapeutic agents directly to the liver through a catheter placed in the hepatic artery.

Hereditary nonpolyposis colon cancer (HNPCC): A hereditary disease resulting in the formation of one to five precancerous polyps at an early age.

Hyperplastic polyp: A noncancerous polyp.

I

Ileus: The time period when the intestines are inactive after major surgery.

Image-guided radiation therapy (IGRT): The use of frequent imaging during a course of radiation therapy to improve the precision and accuracy of the delivery of treatment.

Incentive spirometer: A plastic device that patients blow into after surgery to keep their lungs expanded and prevent pneumonia.

Incision: The surgical site where the actual cutting was performed during surgery.

Inflammatory bowel disease (IBD): A disease characterized by inflammation of the lining or the entire wall of the colon.

Inflammatory polyp: Growths which occur with acute or chronic inflammation.

Intensity modulated radiation therapy (IMRT): A mode of high-precision radiotherapy that uses computer-controlled linear accelerators to deliver precise radiation doses to a tumor or specific areas within the tumor.

Internal radiation therapy: A form a treatment in which a source of radiation is placed inside the body.

Intraoperative radiation therapy (IORT): An intensive radiation treatment that delivers a concentrated beam of radiation to tumors as they are located during surgery.

Intravenous: Refers to inside the vein. Many medications are given this way.

J

Jaundice: A yellowing color of the skin or eyes as a result of a rise in the bilirubin level.

K

KRAS: A protein involved in cell division. The official name is v-Ki-ras2 Kirsten rat sarcoma viral oncogene homolog.

L

Laparoscopic surgery: Surgery performed using small incisions and small instruments.

Linear accelerator (LINAC): A device that creates the X-ray beams used during radiation therapy.

Liver: The largest organ in the abdominal cavity; involved in the processing of blood toxins, glucose metabolism, and the digestion of food.

Low anterior resection: Major operation performed to treat rectal cancer.

Lymph nodes: Pea-size glands located throughout the body and involved in fighting off infection.

Lynch syndrome: A rare inherited condition that increases your risk of colon and other cancers.

M

Magnetic resonance imaging (MRI) scan: A specialized X-ray test using electrons to create detailed pictures of the human body.

Malignant tumor: A tumor that is cancerous and can spread to other parts of the body.

Metastasis: The spreading of a cancerous growth to organs in the body.

Minimally invasive surgery: Surgery performed using small incisions, fiber-optic cameras, and small surgical instruments.

Mucosa: The inner layer of cells lining an organ.

Muscularis propria: The muscle layer of cells surrounding the mucosa in an organ.

Mutation: A DNA change in a gene resulting in an abnormal functioning and, potentially, disease.

N

Nadir: The point at which blood cell counts are at their lowest point after chemotherapy treatment.

Nasogastric tube: A long, clear plastic tube inserted into a patient's stomach during and after surgery to drain any fluid collecting in the stomach.

Neoadjuvant chemotherapy: Chemotherapy that is given before the primary or main treatment.

Neuropathy: A disease or abnormality of the nervous system.

Neutropenia: Describes the state of a very low white blood cell count.

O

Oncologist: A doctor specializing in the medical treatment of cancer.

P

Palliative treatment: Treatment aimed at slowing a disease rather than curing it.

Pathologist: A doctor trained specifically to examine tissue and perform autopsies.

Patient-controlled anesthesia (PCA): A type of postoperative pain control involving the continuous infusion of intravenous narcotic medicine.

Pelvic exenteration: A radical surgical treatment that removes all organs from the pelvic cavity. The urinary bladder, urethra, rectum, and anus are removed.

Pericolonic fat: The fat immediately adjacent to the colon wall.

Peutz-Jeghers syndrome: An inherited disease resulting in the formation of numerous benign colorectal polyps at an early age.

Polyp: An abnormal growth that can occur in any organ, especially the colon. Polyps can be benign or malignant.

Port: A small medical appliance that is installed beneath the skin. A catheter connects the port to a vein. Under the skin, the port has a septum through which chemotherapy drugs can be injected.

Positron emission tomography (PET) scan: An imaging test that shows how tissues and organs are functioning

Postoperative ileus: A disruption of the normal propulsive ability of the gastrointestinal tract after surgery.

R

Radiation oncologist: A doctor trained to perform radiation therapy on patients for the treatment of cancer.

Radiofrequency ablation: A medical procedure in which a tumor is removed using heat generated from the high frequency alternated current.

Radiologist: A doctor trained to perform and read all X-rays.

Rectum: The last six inches of colon leading to the anus.

Recurrence: The return of a cancer during the follow-up period after the initial treatment has been carried out.

Red blood cells: Cells circulating in the body involved in the metabolism of oxygen and iron.

Resection: To remove surgically.

S

Screening: Periodic testing for a specific disease.

Serosa: The outer layer of cells surrounding any organ.

Sessile: Describes the shape of a polyp as being flat and broad based.

Sigmoid colon: The part of the colon starting at the end of the left, or descending, colon and connecting to the rectum.

Sigmoidoscopy: A procedure using a lighted scope to examine the sigmoid colon and rectum.

Snare: A wire device used to remove polyps from the colon during a colonoscopy.

Spleen: The organ located beneath the left rib cage and involved in the immune system's ability to fight infection.

Staging: The process of classifying the extent to which a diagnosed cancer has spread.

Stoma: A surgically created opening in the large intestine that allows the passage of feces into a pouch or other collection device.

Stomatitis: Inflammation of the mucous lining of any of the structures in the mouth.

Stool DNA test: Designed to identify recognizable DNA markers in cells that are continually shed from the lining of the colon and into stool.

Submucosa: The layer of cells just beneath the inner lining, or mucosa, of an organ.

Subtotal colectomy: An operation involving removal of 90 percent of the colon.

T

Tenesmus: The sensation of pressure in the rectum immediately after having a bowel movement.

Three-dimensional conformal radiation therapy (3D-CRT): Treatment that uses computers and special imaging techniques to show the size, shape and location of a tumor.

Thrombocytopenia: Any disorder in which there is an abnormally low amount of platelets.

Total colectomy: An operation performed to remove the entire colon.

Transanal exision: Surgery for rectal cancer that spares the anus and leaves the sphincter intact.

Transrectal ultrasound: An Imaging test using sound waves to evaluate a tumor in the rectum.

Transverse colon: The portion of the colon connecting the right and left colon segments.

Tubular: Referring to the tubelike shape of cells in some polyps.

Tubulovillous: A type of polyp that grows in the colon and other places in the gastrointestinal tract and sometimes in other parts of the body.

Tumor: A tissue growth that can be benign or malignant.

Tumor markers: Substances found in the blood, urine, or body tissues that can be elevated if caner is present.

Turcot's syndrome: An inherited disease resulting in the formation of numerous colorectal polyps.

U

Ulcerative colitis: A serious chronic inflammatory disease of the large intestine and rectum characterized by recurrent episodes of abdominal pain, fever, chills. and profuse diarrhea.

Ultrasound test: An X-ray or imaging test using sound waves to analyze an organ.

V

Villous: Refers to the microscopic description of a particular polyp.

Virtual colonoscopy: A medical imaging procedure that uses X-rays and computers to produce two- and three-dimensional images of the colon from the lowest part, the rectum, all the way to the lower end of the small intestine.

Index

About the Authors

Paul Ruggieri, M.D., is a board-certified general surgeon in private practice in southeastern Massachusetts. Dr. Ruggieri received his medical degree from the Georgetown University School of Medicine in Washington, D.C. Dr. Ruggieri completed his surgical internship and residency at Barnes Hospital, Washington University School of Medicine, St. Louis, Missouri.

After his medical training, Dr. Ruggieri joined the Army and was stationed at the U.S. Army hospital in Fort Polk, Louisiana. During his time in the military, he rose to the rank of major, received the Army Commendation and Meritorious Service Medals, and became the chief of the department of surgery. In 1995, Dr. Ruggieri entered a private surgical practice near Nashville, Tennessee. In 1998, he returned to his native New England to join a surgical group in southeastern Massachusetts.

Dr. Ruggieri is a fellow in the American College of Surgeons and is a member of the Society of American Gastrointestinal Endoscopic Surgeons. He is also the co-author of *A Simple Guide to Thyroid Disorders* (Addicus Books, 2010) and is the author of *The Surgery Handbook: A Guide to Understanding Your Operation* (Addicus Books, 1999).

Addison R. Tolentino, M.D., is a medical oncologist and hematologist with the Avera Medical Group, Oncology and Hematology, in Sioux Falls, South Dakota. He is board certified with the American Board of Internal Medicine in three subspecialties: medical oncology, hematology, and internal medicine.

Dr. Tolentino is also a member of the American Society of Clinical Oncologists, the American College of Physicians, and the American Society of Hematology.

Dr. Tolentino is a graduate of the University of the Philippines College of Medicine in Manila. He completed his internal medicine residency at Montefiore Medical Center, Albert Einstein College of Medicine in Bronx, New York. He completed a fellowship in medical oncology and hematology from Stony Brook University, State University of New York, in Stony Brook, New York.

Consumer Health Titles from Addicus Books

Visit our online catalog at www.AddicusBooks.com

To Order Books:
Visit us online at: www.AddicusBooks.com
Call toll free: (800) 352-2873

For discounts on bulk purchases, call our Special Sales
Department at (402) 330-7493.
Or email us at: info@Addicus Books.com

Addicus Books
P.;O. Box 45327
Omaha, NE 68145

Addicus Books is dedicated to publishing consumer health books
that comfort and educate.